THE ZERO CALORIE DIET

THE ZERO CALORIE DIET

How To Eat Better - Or Not At All!

MICHAEL FINE, MD

This book could not have been published without the help of Kim McHale, who brought design sense, web skills, and common sense to the project. I had help from both Michael Pollen and Marion Nestle, and over the years, from the nutritionists Karen Zengari, Elena Stone, and MaryLou Hixson, but the opinions expressed here are the sole responsibility of the author. No book or author can replace the advice of a person's personal physician: please consult your physician before changing your diet or beginning to fast.

To the people of Pawtucket, Scituate, and Foster, Rhode Island, who let me earn a living for 17 years seeing my friends all day long, and who taught me everything that is in this book.

Rules of The Zero Calorie Diet

Don't eat. Drink. Replace salt. Forget starch.

Don't eat much of anything. You don't need to.

Only 2 food groups from now on: protein and vegetables. Starch is history.

Ignore almost anything the FDA or USDA tells you. Information from the Institute of Medicine is more reliable, but is still filled with the biases of a materialistic culture.

Share meals. It's the taste, not the volume.

If you think you are hungry, you are probably thirsty. Drink.

Drink all day long.

Don't leave food out. You'll eat it.

If you want to reduce eating suddenly, take more salt than usual, and drink plenty of fluids.

Fasting is OK once in a while. It's penitence for being part of a culture that is off the tracks.

Stamp out greed.

Contents

Introduction

In March of 2003, just before the shock-and-awe bombings of Baghdad and the US invasion of Iraq, I began what was to become a 3 week fast.

There was no logical reason for me to fast. I had done no preparation, and didn't know anything about how to go about a long fast, other than the little bits of physiology and metabolism I knew as a family physician. It wasn't a protest fast, like those undertaken by Gandhi or IRA detainees, designed to rally support for a cause. I was upset about the invasion, to be sure, but I kept my choice to myself – no press releases, no interviews, no sending thousands of emails. The left in the US had failed to stop the drumbeats leading to war, which by then was already inevitable, and I am not a public figure, no one would have cared about the fast of an unknown family doctor in rural Rhode Island. It wasn't a weight control fast – I was a little heavy, to be sure, and didn't exercise enough, but I know, and knew, that there are better ways to lose weight, safer ways, and ways that let you keep weight off over the long term.

If anything, it was a personal fast, for perspective, and perhaps, for penitence. We were about to shower bombs on a small foreign country, seeking a conquest that was only about ego and oil and, I feared we were about to kill 100,000 people, while most Americans, the rest of the world, and me, my friends and family, just stood by and watched. 100,000 people. I didn't know what, if anything more, I could have done to stop the invasion. I had written a couple of letters, and a couple of OpEDs. I had gone, once or twice, to small protests outside the Federal Building in Providence. I talked to all my patients, and encouraged everyone who thought war was a bad idea to write letters, or demonstrate themselves. But I could have done more, and I could have worked harder, and if I and people like me had done more than just going through the motions, daintily retracing our steps of a dance from 35 years before, perhaps we would have stopped what was plainly insane. Perhaps.

One morning I awoke and just started fasting.

I had fasted before. Jews fast once a year, on Yom Kippur, also a time for prayer and repentance. That's a 25 hour fast, and it is absolute – no food or water – but it has always been pretty easy for me. I had done a couple of two and three day fasts, which were just to clear my head. I always liked the clean feeling I had after the Yom Kippur fast, the clear headedness, the sweetness of everything I ate or drank as soon as it was over, so from time to time, I'd try a fast during the year. And I have a family history of fasting. My grandfather, Abraham Lieb Gross, was a vegetarian and faster of many years experience, who used to dye his hair white with the lemon juice he put on his tossed salads, and who died from a heart attack after getting TB, which he contracted after becoming malnourished as a result of fasting. He was a frequenter of the Catskills Yiddish health food nut resorts, where crazy Jewish immigrants from the Lower East Side, Brooklyn and the Bronx in their fifties used to go, circa 1938, to eat yoghurt or nothing, take steam baths, play pinochle, and listen to lectures by socialists, Zionists, bundists, labor Zionists, strong men, and cabbalists, all of whom really believed that eating right (or not eating), and eating so much fiber that you'd have stools that floated, was the pathway to social justice, peace in the Middle East, eternal life and youth. So fasting, and some degree of health nuttiness, was clearly in my genes, though I had somehow managed to avoid most of the other craziness associated with that tradition as it came down to my generation – yoga, high colonics and obsessions with yeast and crystals.

And I knew that fasting had its risks, at least on paper. I had gone to medical school in Cleveland, where an endocrinologist and professor of medicine (and, apparently, a man descended from the same crazed Yiddish vegetarian health nuts that I am) supposedly made himself a large fortune by dreaming up very low calorie diets, to help the very plump ladies from Shaker Heights shed their extra pounds. In those days, they would put the obese folks from Shaker Heights in the hospital, arguing (correctly, it turned out) that medical treatment for obesity was indicated, because morbid obesity, defined as being 100 lbs. or more over ideal body weight or having a Body Mass Index (BMI) of 40 or higher, was just as dangerous to your health as having a heart attack or kidney failure. What was the medical treatment? Getting to sit in your room, and drink one specially concocted (and proprietary, ergo the big fortuna) 300 to 400 calorie protein drink a day, on the theory that, as your body broke down and digested its own tissues in order to get enough energy to keep you breathing and your heart pumping, the protein would keep your muscles from breaking down, so you would only break down fat. (Incorrect, and patently absurd, as it turned out – but more about that later).

As a medical student, I had the opportunity to care for one of these plump patients, and being diligent, and not overly convinced by the need to keep these people in the hospital, looked up and read all the world's literature at the time – about 4 papers—on the subject, only to find the reason for hospitalization. The reason? The incidence of sudden cardiac death from prolonged fasting was then reported to be 10 percent.[1] [2] 10 Percent! Talk about patent absurdities! Fearing sudden

1 Brown JM, Yetter JF, Spicer MJ, Jones JD. JAMA. Cardiac complications of protein-sparing modified fasting.1978 Jul 14;240(2):120-2.

2 Sours HE, Frattali VP, Brand CD, Feldman RA, Forbes AL, Swanson RC, Paris AL. Sudden death asociated with very low calorie weight reduction regimens. Am J Clin Nutr. 1981 Apr;34(4):453-61

death, we put people in the hospital, forgetting, of course, that no hospital has ever prevented a cardiac sudden death just by being a hospital. (The theory at the time was, if you had a sudden cardiac death from a prolonged fast, at least there would be people in the hospital who could resuscitate you. But that was before we had all figured out that few people who have a sudden cardiac death actually get successfully resuscitated and live to tell the tale, in or out of the hospital. So much for science. Long live big fortunas.)

So we put people in the hospitals to fast, understanding that the risk of sudden cardiac death from fasting was about 10 percent, and somehow missing the point that the risk of our therapy – fasting—approached the risk of the disease – morbid obesity. Who said medicine is science or even public health?

I, on the other hand, started fasting as penitence for a war that hadn't begun, using a time tested way of creating public sympathy for a cause I hadn't told anyone about, knowing only that there was a ten percent chance of dying from the fast itself, and having no idea how to go about fasting.

But oh. I knew one more thing, which is the difference between eating and drinking. Eating is no big deal. The standard story is that you need to eat about 2000 calories a day (calories, being a measure of heat energy, allow us to compare different foods in terms of how much energy they contain, and how likely they are to add weight to the body, which takes all extra energy sources, and reprocesses them, storing them as fat). The body usually has lots of extra energy in storage, so if you don't eat for a few days – the body just takes some stored fat off the shelf, turns it into energy, and you lose a little weight. Not eating is really no big deal, at least for a couple of days.

Not drinking, on the other hand, is a hugely big deal, and very different from fasting per se. The body is always losing fluid, whether you are trying to or not. You lose fluid in sweat, and you lose fluid in urine, and you even lose fluid in stool. Because fluid is the vehicle for getting rid of chemical wastes that become toxic if not eliminated, you need to constantly replace fluid, by at least 2 quarts a day. Go a day without drinking, and you become dehydrated. In a day. Go two days without drinking anything, and you actually start to go into shock. Go more than three to five days without drinking, and your kidneys start to shut down, and in no more than about 2 weeks, and most often less than 4 weeks, you go into coma, and die. So fasting, if it means not eating, might be hard, but fasting, if it means not drinking, can quickly become lethal. I was penitent, but I wasn't suicidal. A fast for me was going to be a food fast. I'd drink some fruit juice, because, while I was dreading the deaths we would cause in the war yet to

4

come, I wasn't ready to immolate myself in the public, or even private, square.

Remembering the Yom Kippur fast, and suffering the usual American over-inflated ego sense of being invulnerable, I figured I'd blow through fasting for a few days or even a few weeks, and would fast until either we gave up the invasion of Iraq, or until the bombs started falling. My family would look at me a little weird, when I sat at the dinner table and had a glass of orange juice while they ate hot dogs and pizza. I'd drink my fruit juice, repent our coming sins, clean out my system, try to hold a mystical finger in the dike, hoping to use magic to prevent a holocaust because nothing else seemed to be working - and would lose a little weight in the bargain. I'd work normally - see patients, go to meetings, round at the hospital, write and think and answer emails. Fasting, but no big deal.

Day One. No big deal. A little lightheaded.

Day Two. More lightheaded. Headache at the end of the day.

Day Three. Lightheaded on arising. Lethargic by 10 am. Can barely stand up at the end of the day.

Day Four. Like day three, only worse.

Day Five. Still worse. Don't think I can do this any more.

A little physiology intruded here. The body, when it starts to fast, flips a switch, and goes from what's called the *fed* state to what's called the *fasting* state. Existing on your own fat stores for energy – breaking down your own tissues to support heartbeat, breathing and thinking (which actually consumes lots of energy, at least for some of us) – a process called catabolism – actually takes a little time. You have to manufacture new enzymes to support this process, and that takes 12 to 36 hours. Once you flip the switch, your body actually functions pretty well on the alternative fuel source – your own tissues-- your energy comes back, your breath smells sweet (because of a process called ketosis) and your head clears – but the transition itself can be very difficult, because for a time you have little or no real energy source – no food, and no energy from your own tissues.

So the third day didn't make sense. The switch from the fed state to the fasting state should have been over by the middle of the second day. Why did I feel so bad in the middle of the third day? I could barely stand up, and barely listen to patients who were talking to me. I found an empty exam room, and took 10 minutes to lay down on an examination table – and then struggled to keep my eyes open and my head up as I talked to patients the rest of the day. At home that night, all I could do was sleep – no energy for paperwork, email, or writing. What was going on?

The fourth day was no better. I didn't think I could fast and work.

By the fifth day I was ready to quit.

I don't remember what took me to my first cup of bouillon. I think it was just there – an old bottle of bouillon cubes kept for making chicken stock. I was still trying not to eat, but my resolve was getting weaker. A cup of bouillon – not fruit juice, but not eating either. At least it wasn't solid food.

It took about a minute to heat a cup of water in the microwave, unwrap, and plop the cube into the hot water, stir, and drink the concoction. I still remember how salty it tasted, and how good it was, in the way the taste of all food comes alive after a fast. I think I followed it with a glass of plain water, rinsed out the glass, and prepared to drag myself back to work.

But then, an amazing thing happened. Suddenly, without warning, my brain came back. My headache cleared. Energy, back to what it had been. Hunger, gone. Lethargy, gone. Suddenly, I was back to my normal self, in the middle of a five day fast. I went back to the kitchen, and found the bottle of bouillon cubes, so I could look at the nutritional information on the label, expecting that bouillon cubes were somehow loaded with sugar, because everything in US packaged food is loaded with corn starch and fructose. No corn starch. No sugar. 10 calories! Just flavoring and 1000 milligrams of sodium. 1000 milligrams of sodium!!! It was all salt.

I would later make sense of the physiology and metabolism. You feel bad when you fast because of salt and fluid metabolism, and not because of calories, not because of carbohydrate and sugar. Fasting makes you dehydrated, unless you carefully attend to your salt and fluid intake.

But the flip side, that lots of what we eat has nothing to do with what we need, would only occur to me later. Worse, the realization that lots of illness and expense – heart disease, diabetes, high cholesterol, high blood pressure, stroke and blindness – is caused by what we eat, and that we eat what we eat because someone profits by our doing that, would only occur to me much later indeed.

Working with Karen Zangari and Elena Stone, nutritionist colleagues, I would later work out how to fast without feeling bad. Sometime after that, thinking about American medicine, a wealth extraction system build on profit, instead of a health care system, I came to understand that eating in America is also about profit, and not nourishment or sustenance. The extent to which our lives focus on activities that create profit for others got me thinking about pushing away from the table together, so we can all think about living lives that matter, instead buying what someone else has to sell.

Those two ideas – that we can learn lots about how to eat from fasting, and most of what we feed ourselves is there to create profit for others instead of sustenance for ourselves and the people around us, led to The Zero Calorie Diet.

First disclaimer. The title is something of a come-on, to make you think about how advertising works in your life, and gets you to buy things and do things because the advertising tells you to do it, or is pitched to draw your attention to a promise that might not be real. It is not possible to both eat Zero Calories and have a long and productive life. Thirty years ago, a "Breatharian" named Wiley Brooks in California (ah, California) supposedly made hundreds of thousands of dollars giving seminars, telling people how they could live on air. His empire fell apart when a smart reporter followed him and caught him going into a fast food joint, though he will still sell you his secret for $25 million, up front. In cash. Non refundable. Ain't capitalism grand?

Truth be told, The Zero Calorie Diet isn't a really a diet after all. The Zero Calorie Diet is a fast, which no normal person is going to do more than a few days. Diets don't work, anyway. People lose weight on a diet, which they stick to for a few weeks or months, then slip back into their old eating and exercise habits, and the weight comes back with the old habits.

But fasts don't work either, as a life style, because fasts aren't sustainable over time. Fasts work pretty well as a way to draw a distinction between your normal life and the time you are fasting, and that distinction is sometimes helpful getting you to look at how you are living, and sometimes helps you decide to change how you are living. The Zero Calorie Diet is just that, a way of living. Living with few calories, because having thought about what happens to the body during a fast, we learn about how to live with less food, and learn a little more about how to live with each other, instead of living on one another's backs. The Zero Calorie Diet is also a way of thinking - thinking about what people really need from each other, which is time, love, and acceptance, instead of thinking about false needs, irrational fears, arrogance, and artificial or inflated desires, inserted into our lives by someone with something to sell. We got sold on the invasion of Iraq because we weren't thinking clearly. Let's not get fooled again.

There is an underlying purpose to The Zero Calorie Diet beyond helping you understand how to eat and how not to eat. The cost of health care in the US is crippling our economy, and ruining our communities. We spend about 2.3 trillion dollars a year on medical services – twice as much as the average of the other industrialized countries in the world – and have population health that ranks our health care system only 37th to 101st in the world. We waste about half of what we spend – about $1 trillion a year – on unnecessary services. But much of the rest is spent on treating illnesses – heart disease, diabetes, and even some cancers – that we have caused ourselves. We cause much of the illness and premature death in the US by an economic system that puts profit before the public health, and by bad public policy that encourages the bad actors in our economic system to make more by selling more, regardless of its value. Our public policy subsidizes growing the wrong food, doesn't adequately stop companies from putting the wrong chemicals in our air and water, and rewards people and companies that help people spend time in the wrong ways, doing less physical work, and spending more time sitting alone on the couch in front of one kind of screen or another. We are being crippled by public policies that promote growing too much of the wrong foods – mostly corn and wheat -- and by a culture of greed that allows companies to profit by making and selling packaged food products that are bad for the people who consume them. We are causing disease by creating a culture that pushes people to eat because they are anxious and alone, not because they need nutritional sustenance. (A culture that promotes sitting in front of the TV instead of being outside, working together with friends, doesn't help.) If The Zero Calorie Diet can help us understand how to change what we eat and not eat, and how much we exercise, and how to spend more time together, even just a little bit, the public health effects of this book are likely to dwarf the public health effects of all my years of practicing family medicine, and spouting public health policy.

My very clear bias is that we have caused most of the illness we then have to pay to treat by creating a culture that makes people anxious enough to eat what they don't need, and allowing an economy in which other people profit from all that useless eating.

This book owes a tremendous amount to the work of Marion Nestle, Brian Minsink, and Michael Pollan. Marion Nestle is a nutritionist who has carefully traced the influence of the food industry on what we eat. Brian Minsink, trained as a marketer and evolved into a very smart food psychologist, has worked for years to tease out what makes us eat, and how the food industry plays on those cues. Michael Pollan is a journalist who put together and popularized some of the basic connections, and fundamental disconnects, between profit, nutrition, economy, and health. Pollan's simple conclusion – "eat food, mostly plants, not too much" - is at the heart of most of the advice given here. Pollan tells us what to do. I try to sketch out what not to do, and how not to do it.

Second Disclaimer. Talk to your doctor before modifying your own diet. Everyone is different. And interesting.

Part I - The Zero Calorie Diet

The Zero Calorie Diet

The Zero Calorie Diet isn't a diet. It's a fast. Anything with zero calories is a fast. A diet is something provided or experienced regularly, food and drink regularly provided or consumed, or a regimen of eating and drinking sparingly so as to reduce one's weight.[3] When you go on The Zero Calorie Diet, you aren't taking anything in, regularly or irregularly. You will lose weight. But I make no claims about the long term benefits of The Zero Calorie Diet for your health and well-being. Carried on long enough, The Zero Calorie Diet won't just reduce your weight. Over time, if you do it long enough, The Zero Calorie Diet will kill you, despite what the Breatharians claim.

But weight loss is not the reason for going on The Zero Calorie Diet, since no diet works for weight loss over the long term. As any good nutritionist (and a lot of bad ones, though I never met a nutritionist I didn't like) will tell you, the way to lose weight is to change your lifestyle, to change how you look at food, nutrition, sustenance, relationships and the world. That's what The Zero Calorie Diet will do for you. The Zero Calorie Diet will put you in the driver's seat.

The Zero Calorie Diet itself is pretty simple. No food. No calories. Drink plenty of liquids, some with enough sodium to replace your normal sodium losses -- or 1.5 to 2 grams of sodium a day -- which you can get by drinking fruit juices, an athlete's drink, an artificially colored drink like Gatorade (all of which are usually loaded with calories), or bouillon, which is the most efficient way to replace sodium over all. I like the combination of a cup or two of bouillon, and 10 to 15 eight ounce glasses of a clear liquid, which I often drink as decaffeinated tea or water, with a half ounce or so of fruit juice in it, for flavor.

I exercise during The Zero Calorie Diet for a couple of hours a day. I'm into the third day of a three day fast as I write this, and I've been spending 2-4 hours a day cutting and bringing in firewood – pretty strenuous stuff. I think, but can't prove, that exercise is actually what makes fasting safe, because exercise sends genetic and hormonal signals to the muscles to grow and strengthen, which I think, but can't prove, counteracts the breakdown of all tissues, called catabo-

---

3 http://www.merriam-webster.com/dictionary/diet. 12/9/2008 7:31 AM

lism, that otherwise occurs during fasting. I think, but can't prove, that the failure to exercise is what explains the significant number of cardiac sudden deaths in people who did the old 300 calorie protein sparing fasts, from the 1970s and 80s, and the lack of reported sudden death in people after bariatric surgery.

Somewhere between 12 and 36 hours on The Zero Calorie Diet, you'll get foggy for a few hours, and feel like lying down. Go ahead. Lie down. The fogginess will pass. That fogginess is what happens when your body runs out of energy from glucose and other forms of stored sugars, just before it reprocesses enough energy from fat to make the body run well as a machine. After the fogginess passes, you will notice two things. First, that you have stopped being hungry. You aren't dying for food. If you get a little "why don't I get up and have an xxxx (high calorie snack)" feeling, go and drink a glass of water or tea, and the feeling will go away.

The second thing you will notice is mental clarity, which happens on the third or fourth day. Instead of feeling foggy and tired, you will become mentally clear and full of energy, as if you have been given new life.

One important observation. If you eat 4000 calories on the day you stop fasting, and then resume an 1800 calorie diet when you've learned you need 1200, you'll gain 2/3 of a pound quickly, and will keep gaining. If you start eating 1200 calories, then you won't regain the weight you lost by fasting. The number of calories eaten and burned in 1 day doesn't matter, which is why diets don't work. It's the number of calories eaten and burned in your lifetime that matters. Unfortunately, every calorie counts – every single bloody calorie contributes to your current weight. It's not fair, but it is true.

Any weight you lose in The Zero Calorie Diet is actually either burned fat or burned carbohydrate or burned protein. It's not water. People who diet lose water in the first few days of the diet because they reduce their sodium intake suddenly, and it takes a few days for the kidneys to figure out what's going on, and start to hold on to sodium, which brings the blood volume back to what it should be. (More on the physiology of blood volume and sodium retention later.) The loss of water in traditional diets is what happens because blood volume shrinks when you lose sodium, because you need a certain amount of sodium to keep fluid in your veins. But people on The Zero Calorie Diet replace their sodium as they fast, and so they can maintain their effective blood volume and keep the normal amount of fluid in their bodies. You won't lose water on The Zero Calorie Diet. Just real weight – just fat, carbohydrate stores, and muscle.
Should you try The Zero Calorie Diet? I think so, but not for the usual reasons

people try diets, which usually don't work anyway. Try The Zero Calorie Diet because it will help you learn that you really don't need to eat, at least not in the short term. The Zero Calorie Diet is a way to look at what you have been doing, how you have been living, and what and how you have been eating. It gives you the space to discover what it is you really need from food, which in our culture is not much. Food is a little necessary in the long term, but is not that important day to day or moment to moment. Drinking fluid, and replacing sodium, that's what is important day to day and moment to moment. Eating is a good excuse to have or share a meal with people you know and love, which to most of us, is what really matters. Not calories, or protein, not fat. The people you know and love.

But more important, try The Zero Calorie Diet because it works. Yes, you'll lose a little weight, but there are easier, more sensible ways of losing weight than fasting (or dieting!!). More important, you'll finish a three and a half day fast, feeling great, and realize you could keep going if you wanted to. The amazing thing about The Zero Calorie Diet is that it teaches you that you can live without food for a few days or a few weeks. As long as you keep drinking, and replace your sodium losses, you learn that you won't go crazy if you don't eat. You'll learn that all the messages coming into your brain from your environment, from the TV, the internet, from magazines and billboards and the radio and a lifetime of subliminal messages in a culture that seems totally focused on both getting you to eat anything and everything and getting you to buy stuff that will either help you stop eating, or fixing the damage you've done to yourself by eating – that whole Halleluiah chorus of messages, can be ignored. You'll learn you don't really need to eat right away, ever, and you'll learn that you can feel as good not eating as you do eating, and maybe even better.

That freedom, the freedom from the compulsion to eat, is a very powerful force. First, you learn you need to drink, but not eat. Then you learn you don't need to shop. Then you start looking at the world in a different way. Do we need to live like this? Did we need to invade Iraq?

How long should you do The Zero Calorie Diet? Do The Zero Calorie Diet only until you are comfortable that eating isn't what's important day to day, drinking is, and only until you are really ready to break bread (or better, break open a watermelon), with people you love. Then, when things seem stuck, when you feel like you aren't seeing things as they are, like you aren't being effective in getting done what you want to get done, or being with whom you want to be, do The Zero Calorie Diet again.

Don't do The Zero Calorie Diet to lose weight. Do The Zero Calorie Diet to draw a distinction between the time when you are not eating and your normal life, to give yourself a place to stand, so you can look at the relationships between your food, your eating, the people who produce the food, the people who profit from the food, the people who tell you what you need, your sense of what is important, your life and the world around you, and ask yourself whether it all makes sense.

14

$$\boxed{\text{Lean}}$$

Some of the lessons from The Zero Calorie Diet have to do with how to look at your eating habits and beliefs, and some have to do with your habits, beliefs, choices and actions in general. Some lessons are more specific: how many calories you really need. How long most of us can go without eating. The role sodium and fluid play in how you feel when you eat less. The obsolescence of the three food group meal, and in particular, the obsolescence of starch in the diets of Americans.

These lessons are lessons about how to think about food, nutrition, eating, and sustenance when you are not following The Zero Calorie Diet, which ought to be most of the time.

A central question, which we should address together now, is the purpose of food, and eating, and the meaning of health.

I come from a profession that profits by frightening people about the risks to them that come from their habits, choices, genetics, and destiny. That is, the health care marketplace in general, and doctors in particular, leverage a particular world view, that not everyone shares. That world view, which might be called the healthism strain of logical positivism, operates from the following set of beliefs, which it assumes everyone shares: the only thing that matters in human life is living as long as possible. It may be possible to live forever or at least for a very long time, if you eat the foods we tell you to eat, have the experiences we tell you to have, avoid the experiences we tell you to avoid, and take the drugs we tell you to take.

Of course, almost none of that dogma is true.

As we discuss food, nutrition, eating, and sustenance, it is important to identify how those biases influence our thinking and talking about eating and not eating. There is a huge bias around weight, for example, that is connected to much discussion around food, nutrition, eating, and sustenance. The health care marketplace wants you to believe that you will live longer, feel better, look better, even have more and better sex (as if more and better sex were a central value of the human experience) if you weigh less. Many of those claims have some truth to them, if you believe that living as long as possible, feeling better, looking better (with looking better usually being defined by tastemakers who have products to sell) and having more and better sex, are values for you, and are the things that matter to you, the values you want to build your life around.

But those things may not matter to you. It's okay if you want to smoke and drink and sit in the park all day, drinking beer and playing chess – understanding you have a higher risk of dying at 45 than someone who doesn't do those things – but on the other hand, someone who doesn't do those things also has a real but smaller risk of dying at 45, and perhaps, dying after 45 years of not as much fun. It's okay not to take your medicine if you have high blood pressure and just hate taking medicine, as long as you understand the risks you take of stroke and heart disease, risks associated with untreated high blood pressure. It's your life, and the only person who can choose what to do with it is you.

And even if living a long time, looking at a certain definition of fit, (and having more and better sex) does matter to you, it is also important to understand that experience is not predictable. That is, you may learn to weigh less, and not feel better, not live longer, and not have more or better sex, so before you change your life, it is important to understand that change may not bring the rewards you want, if those are the rewards you want.

To me, that is the meaning of lean.

That is, at one level, I know that two thirds of Americans are overweight or actually obese, as we define overweight and obesity, and 31 percent are actually overweight, that we have an epidemic of diabetes, cancer, heart disease and stroke, which is fueled by Americans being overweight, that those diseases cost $78 billion a year or more, and if people weren't obese, we'd have that money to spend on education, housing, the environment and public safety, which turn out to be the kind of programs that make people feel better, and actually live longer.[4] [5]   And there is growing medical evidence that being really lean, having a body mass index of 20 or less which is really, really thin, is associated with less disease and longer life spans.[6] [7]

---

4 Ogden CL, Carroll MD, Curtin LR, McDowell MA, Tabak CJ, Flegal KM. Prevalence of overweight and obesity in the United States, 1999-2004. JAMA. 2006 Apr 5;295(13):1549-55

5 Finkelstein, EA, Fiebelkorn, IC, Wang, G. National medical spending attributable to overweight and obesity: How much, and who's paying? Health Affairs 2003;W3;219–226.

6 Fontana L, Klein S. Aging, adiposity, and calorie restriction. JAMA. 2007 Mar 7;297(9):986-94

7 Everitt AV, Le Couteur DG. Life extension by calorie restriction in humans. Ann N Y Acad Sci. 2007 Oct;1114:428-33.

But I'm not sure that being lean, being healthier, and living longer, is what we earthlings want, or should want to do.

So lean, to me, is as much about humility as it is about weight. We know that having all these standards of what and how to be has created a world that is hopelessly complex, a world that is always busy, a world in which change always favors the change agents, a world in which half of the world's population is fed but half of the world's population is desperately poor, a world that returns to war again and again. So lean is about listening as much as it is about eating, or not eating. The idea is to get to a place where everyone matters, and the ideas that we all adopt are the ideas that lead to a time where everyone is nourished, everyone is educated, everyone has the time to do what brings them happiness, and we stop killing one another over nothing.

We're too fat with destructive, manipulative ideas. It's never too late to stop and listen.

Listening, and learning from one another, consumes no calories. That's lean.

Part II - Lessons From The Zero Calorie Diet

Relative Rates

It's buried back there, somewhere before you got to algebra, but after you memorized the multiplication and division tables, in a set of word problems designed to help you learn math. A train leaving Chicago is going to New York and travels at 60 miles an hour. An hour later, an airplane leaving New York takes off, headed for Chicago, and is traveling 500 miles an hour. How long does it take for the plane to reach and fly over the train?

The important thing about the relative rate word problem isn't just knowing the rates, but the answer. It's nice to know how fast a train travels. It's nice to know how fast a plane travels. But to get the answer, you need to know how fast both are traveling at the same time, and know the direction in which each its traveling, so you can find out how long it will take for them to meet.

The most important thing we learn from The Zero Calorie Diet is how the relative rates of different kinds of taking in and losing of nutrients impacts bodily functions, and the size and shape of the body itself.

The trick is to remember to balance what is going out with what is coming in. It is really hard to remember to add up all that is coming in, and really hard to remember to keep track of what is going out. Most people have no idea how many calories they are taking in, how few calories they burn in the course of a normal American life, or how much sodium and water is going out. Keep track of what is going in and what is coming out out, keep control of both to keep them in balance (or make what's coming in less than what's going out, if you want to reduce weight) and all the rest is just arithmetic.

The Zero Calorie Diet simplifies relative rate problems for the body. By removing or limiting intake, it helps us to look at the rate of outgo only, and we can learn how to balance what has to go out and how fast it is going, with what little needs to come in.

Let's think about weight over time. Most people are at or near their ideal body weight about the time they graduate from high school. Starting in their twenties, most people gain a pound or two a year, as they become less active and develop regular eating schedules. A pound or two a year doesn't seem like much.

But over 20 years – by their mid thirties, a pound or two a year has become 40-50 pounds.   Relative rates.

The simplest calculation to see how relative rates work is the calculation of how quickly The Zero Calorie Diet – really taking in zero calories – leads to starvation or malnutrition. Body fat contains 3500 calories per pound. (Protein and carbohydrate contain about 1550 calories per pound). If you are overweight, 25 percent or more of your weight is fat.

So say you are female, 5 foot 4 inches, and weigh 175 pounds. That gives you a body mass index of 30, obese according to all standards.

Now say you start to fast. Say you are used to eating 1500 calories a day, an amount which keeps your weight pretty stable, because you walk an hour a day. Now you stop eating all together.

IF you could lose only body fat and not break down other tissues, you'd lose a pound every 2 1/3 days – or a little more than 12 pounds a month. To get to your ideal body weight, which is about 120 pounds, it would take 4 and a half months, of not eating at all!!

Now, try the same thought experiment, only add in an hour of really strenuous exercise a day. If you can really work hard (which few of us do, for a full hour), you might burn an extra 400 calories a day. At 1900 calories a day, you'd lose a pound every 1.8 days, or almost 15 pounds a month. But it would still take more than 3 1/2 months of fasting for you to get back to your ideal body weight.

Most people think a three or four week fast ought to take you back to Gandhi - like slimness. But few of us understand how much extra weight we carry. And it's only by working out the balance of intake and outgo, the relative rates, that we can understand how that weight got there, and how to make it go away again.

Here's a really simple example of how relative rates impact weight loss or gain by food substitution. Say you love ice cream, and eat a cup of ice cream a day. Three scoops, or about 6 ounces, isn't quite a cup, but still delivers about 500 calories a day. Now say you switch over to watermelon, and start eating a cup of watermelon a day. Tasty, not quite as filling, but still enough to satisfy the urge to nibble. 40 calories. You've dropped 460 calories a day. By dropping 460 calories a day, you lose a pound a week. A pound a week is 52 pounds a year. Just by understanding relative rates, and substituting a calorie spare food for a calorie dense food, you've lost as much in a year as you would in a 4 month fast – only without fasting.

The sodium story is also a story of relative rates, and it's the piece of fasting that has been totally missed by medical experts, who always focus on the impact of glucose and breakdown of fat that occurs when people stop eating. Humans lose about 50mg of sodium an hour through sweat, urine, and in stool, losses which the body reduces – but can't eliminate, when eating stops. In all, we lose 3-4 grams of sodium a day – and as much as 6 to 8 grams if you are working outside on a hot day. That's only possible because food – particularly prepared food - is full of sodium, so you are constantly replacing the sodium you are constantly losing. A cookie has 300 mg of sodium. A hot dog has 1100 mg of sodium. A slice of pizza has 700 mg of sodium. We lose so much sodium, and take in so much sodium with every bite, that we don't notice how much goes in and how much goes out, and don't think about how important sodium is to how we feel.

Now add the impact of relative rates. You fast. The intake of food goes away – but your intake of sodium vanishes as well. Intake vanishes, but you are still losing 2 grams a day. Your body has a mechanism to reduce your losses, but it can't reduce those losses to much less than 600mg a day. The total amount of sodium in your body shrinks, and by the mechanisms I discuss in the next chapter, you start to become dehydrated, and feel terrible. So you start eating again – not because you need the calories, which you probably don't, if, like most Americans, you are carrying some extra weight, but because you need the sodium in the food you eat to maintain your fluid volume. Relative rates.

What we learn from not eating is the relative importance of calories (important for losing or maintaining weight, but not important for how you feel when you are fasting), the relative importance of exercise, which helps you to lose weight if you want to, but might make you lose more weight than you want faster than you want if you are fasting, though it has some extra benefits during fasting we haven't fully discussed yet; and the relative importance of sodium, which you don't even notice in daily life, has no impact on weight, but is the critical factor for how you feel when you eat less.

When you think about fasting, eating or eating less, don't think about what you are eating or not eating. Think about relative rates of consuming, and losing, calories and sodium over time. That's the way to fast and keep functioning, and the way to lose weight successfully and keep it off, and the way to think about how to eat, or not eat, and live well over time.

Once you have thought about the impact of relative rates of consuming and losing calories and sodium, then think about the relative rates of individuals and groups of people, consuming and losing relationship and community, consuming and losing control over the environment, consuming and losing equality and property, consuming and losing our hopes and dreams - and then use that perspective to think about our culture and our future. Are we going together where we should go? Perhaps The Zero Calorie Diet, which lets us look at ourselves when we are not consuming, has something to tell us about who we are and who we can still be.

The Song of Salt and Men

So it's salt, not sugar, that makes you feel bad when you are fasting, and when you are eating less, and salt, not sugar, that drives you to eat more than you need. And salt, not sugar, that will help you not eat, when you realize how people with something to sell have convinced you to eat garbage that's bad for you, so they can make a profit, while your health and wealth go down the tubes.

Let's look at what happens to the body when you stop eating and drinking, in terms of sugar and salt.

The first thing to understand is that the body is programmed to survive changes in the availability of sugar. The second thing to understand is that the bulk of our scientific attention to fasting has been attention to sugar and fat.

The body has lots of energy storage mechanisms, which protect you against feeling bad when you can't (or decide not to) eat. There is a quick release form of glucose, the major sugar used by the body for energy, called glycogen, which is available in the liver, to be used in keeping your blood sugar constant. That gets exhausted by 24 hours of fasting. Then you start to break down fats. Through one of the most elegant mechanisms in the body, which contains lots of complex signaling and switching, by the end of three days of fasting, your body radically reduces the use of glucose for energy, and switches over to the break-down of fat. By the seventh day of a fast, 70 percent of the brain's energy needs comes from the breakdown products of fats, with some glucose being produced from the breakdown of muscle. By seven days, even your basic metabolic rate, the rate at which your heart beats and you breathe, slows, in order to conserve energy, and to keep you feeling well. By 14 days of fasting, 90 percent of your energy requirements come from the breakdown of fat; your metabolism slows by 25 percent; and muscle breakdown, while continuing, slows as well.[8] Less muscle breakdown means less waste for your kidneys to eliminate. Urine flow lessens, so you lose less salt – but you keep losing it anyway.

Compare that to what happens to sodium when you stop eating. The body can't manufacture sodium, so you take in huge amounts – usually five times as much as you lose every day, just for safekeeping. The body only has a certain amount

8 Cahill G. Fuel metabolism in starvation. Ann Rev Nutrition (2006) 26:1-22

of sodium, and it depends on constant eating to keep your sodium level stable, because you are losing sodium every second of the day. (That's why it's a good thing that all food has some sodium, and that's why you are constantly eating.) So the moment you start to fast, and stop taking in sodium by eating, your sodium level starts to drop.

What happens when your sodium level starts to drop is actually quite complex, and somewhat difficult to follow, but basically, you start to go into shock, very gradually. The "extracellular fluid" - the fluid in your arteries and veins that is in tissues, but outside of the cells which make up the living part of tissue, shrinks as the total amount of sodium in your body shrinks, and the impact is immediate. By the time you've lost 2 percent of your extracellular fluid volume, there are measurable impacts on performance and ability.[9] Because sodium is necessary to keep fluid in your arteries and veins, your extracelluar fluid shrinks as the total amount of sodium in the body drops, whether you are drinking plain water or not.

The body's first priority is always to supply blood, which carries oxygen and nutrients, to the brain and other vital organs. To do that, the body always tries to keep the concentration of sodium and other chemicals pretty stable. It's an up-hill battle, though, because you are always losing sodium - you lose more than 1 percent of the sodium that maintains blood volume each day. In the rare event (fasting) that you lose a source of new sodium, your body gets a little confused. It maintains the concentration of sodium, although the only way to do that is to let the actual blood volume shrink, because of the way a physical process called diffusion works. Shock is the name we give to losing 20 percent of that actual blood volume, which is pretty close to what is called extracellular fluid. Once you lose (and don't quickly replace) that 20 percent of extracellular fluid, you can't stand up, can't think, look incredibly pasty, - and are actually near death. Since most of us only have 14 liters or less of extracellular fluid supporting blood volume, that means you go into shock once you lose about three liters – and you lose about 2 ½ liters of fluid every day in urine, and through breathing, sweat and in stool.

Even though you are only losing 1 percent of your total body sodium a day, a little loss of sodium turns into a big loss of extracellular fluid and circulating blood volume, because a very large part of the sodium that's lost comes from that extracelluar fluid. When you are fasting, you lose but don't replace sodium. Most of that sodium comes from the extracellular fluid and circulating blood volume, which shrinks, because of the sodium loss, and you quickly start

---

9 Auerbach: Wilderness Medicine, 5th ed.

to go into shock.

So say you are fasting, but drinking plain water (which has no sodium), or a fluid without much sodium. You lose 1 percent of the important sodium every day, and with it, 2 to 3 liters of fluid. By day two, you've lost 2 percent of your sodium, and now 4 to 6 liters of fluid, even if you are drinking plain water - and you start to notice changes in your ability to think and function. [10] By day three, you've lost 3 percent of your body's total sodium and a very large part of the sodium you use to maintain blood volume and keep your brain functioning, and probably 6 to 8 liters of fluid, which is close to half of your effective blood volume. By day three time, the body is doing everything it can to reduce the loss of sodium – but it can only reduce the loss so much, and you keep getting further and further behind, until you either eat something, which replaces some of that lost sodium, or until your blood volume gets so low you can't stand, and then your kidneys shut down, and you slip into a coma and die.

That's the extreme case.

Now let's run the same scenario, only, instead of fasting, think of what happens if you start eating less.

When you eat less, the essential dynamics are the same – you take in less sodium, and after a few days, your blood volume contracts. That's the bad news. The good news is that food is so chock full of sodium that it takes very little to maintain your blood volume. But if you cut your intake enough, and don't replace the sodium, you will gradually feel it.

How do you feel it? Perhaps you will feel tired or foggy. But more likely, early on, your body will send you a sensation intended to correct the lack the body experiences. What is that sensation? The sensation the body sends when the concentration of sodium in the body starts to drop is one we all know – it's called thirst.

Here's where the story gets interesting. The sensation is thirst, but drinking isn't a perfect fix for the body's problem, which is actually lack of sodium. (Drinking probably provides only a short term boost in effective blood volume, which depends on both sodium and fluid, not fluid itself, to get blood to the brain and vital organs.) So there is compensation. The thirst center and the hunger center in the brain are next to one another, and the body frequently confuses the signals. Instead of drinking, you eat. Sounds like a mistake, right? But it

10 Noble: Textbook of Primary Care Medicine, 3rd ed.2001 Mosby, Inc.

works out perfectly – or perfectly, with one small exception. The blood volume drops, you get thirsty, you confuse hunger and thirst, so you eat. The food has lots of sodium, so the body gets what it needs, the blood volume can expand, and you feel better. Sounds perfect, right?

Perfect except for the side effect of eating in America. Think you are hungry? There are a thousand messages, commercials, food wrappers, and too many leftovers in the refrigerator, and it's a huge trap. You eat, and you get not only sodium, but also calories. The calories reverse the impact of what you had been trying to do by eating less, and the weight never leaves or comes back if it ever comes off. Which is why changing your eating style is so difficult in the good old USA.

So what do we learn about sodium from fasting? People eating less in America need to take sodium into account, and need to remember to replace the sodium they would have taken in, when they eat less. Replace sodium, NOT calories. You want to maintain your sodium intake while dropping your caloric intake if eating less is to be a sustainable lifestyle change.

One quick note about supplementing sodium. Most people know that there is a relationship between salt and high blood pressure, so many will be cautious about supplementing sodium when they eat less. The caution is well founded. About a third of people with high blood pressure have blood pressure that will improve if they reduce the sodium in their diet. Other people with chronic diseases like congestive heart failure and kidney and liver disease need to be very careful about the amount of sodium they ingest. But please note I am not suggesting anyone increase the sodium in their diets. If you eat less by a third, you have dropped your sodium intake by a third. What I am suggesting is only that you keep your sodium intake what it always was.

So a quick rule of thumb. Most Americans take in 3 to 4 grams of sodium a day. If you fast, you need to take in 2 grams of sodium a day to maintain your blood volume, and drink plenty of fluid. If you cut your caloric intake by a third, from say, 1800 to 1200 calories (an intake that makes much more sense for most American adults), understand you'll lose about 1 gram of sodium intake a day, or go from 3 grams to 2 grams. Now, 2 grams is probably plenty of sodium intake, but there is no harm in supplementing by 1 to 2 grams a day, just to make sure you limit the contraction of blood volume, and don't get thirsty, and then hungry, and find yourself eating more again. This "supplementation" is actually only a way to maintain the sodium intake you were used to, and, because it is what you have been taking all along, is not likely to impact your health significantly - it's the same amount of sodium you've been taking in all along.

You know the disclaimer – always talk this over with your own doctor first. But in addition to talking to your doctor, think about how it all works – calories on one side, sodium on the other, sodium loss driving thirst and hunger, and food profiteers hovering all around you, trying to sell you stuff that can only make them rich, and you fat and sick.

We'll talk about how to add salt to a careful diet of mostly plants in chapters about specific foods, to follow.

.

Part III - Why The Zero Calorie Diet Works, But Not As Well As You Think

We Have Met The Enemy, And He Is Us

One of the first things they try to teach you in medical school is that everyone who has ever had a beer, and everyone who is overweight, is a liar.

"They lie about how much they drink. If they say they drink 2 beers a day, assume it's 4 to 6 beers. If they say they drink a pint of scotch a night, assume it's 2 to 3 pints. And everyone who is overweight eats a whole lot more than they admit to. They are all liars."

What a wonderful introduction! How nicely it sets the stage for a lifetime of intimate, collaborative relationships. See where the "doctor is god" complex comes from?

I struggled with that attitude for about 20 years – not that I bought it – I didn't – but because it seemed to explain something I really experienced as I tried to work with people trying to lose weight – struggled with it, until I realized that the only liars are doctors, that I had met the enemy, and the enemy was me.

For years, I worked with a few women who were quite heavy, and were desperate to lose weight. These were good people, solid, loving, honest, committed people, who swore up and down they were sticking to the, first 1800 kcal, and then 1500 kcal diets I, or one of my nutritionist colleagues, gave them. The normal adult is supposed to burn 2000 to 2500 calories a day. For years, though, we've been giving out 1800 calorie diets, on the assumption that everyone is a liar, and if you really need 2500 calories, and we tell you 1800 calories, and you cheat, and really eat 2200 calories, you'll still lose weight – lots of weight, as much as 50 pounds a year.

There was only one problem.

It never worked.

When people didn't lose weight on 1800 calories, the great gods of medicine came up with the only explanation they could possibly imagine – that people who were imperfect, were not perfectly following our perfect advice. They were cheating. Our advice was good. People were bad.

Sometimes we tried an explanation called the metabolic set point, but no one actually believed it. The metabolic set point hypothesis suggests that the body has some kind of magic metabolic regulator that keeps weight at a certain point by slowing the metabolism by about 12 percent once a certain weight is reached, and the slower metabolism means the body burns fewer calories and uses less energy, once you get down to a certain weight, and that means it should be very difficult to lose weight once you hit a certain weight, which differs for every person. Because the so-called regulator is set differently for different people, this is a very difficult hypothesis to test, which means you can't prove the theory, but you can't disprove it either. Great explanation - gets everyone out from under blame and the cheating accusation, and makes a certain kind of physiologic sense - only the metabolic set point argument fails the basic science and math test. You can't slow metabolism to zero. You need to use some energy in the activities of daily life. Once you reduce your intake below a certain point, everyone has to lose weight. The metabolic set point explanation was trotted out for people who never lost weight, despite eating next to nothing. Or not. In our heart of hearts, we all still believe that fat people are lying about what they eat. Despite what we told ourselves about how very good and honest the people who just couldn't lose on the 1500 calories diets we gave them were, and despite those people swearing up and down that they were following our diets to the letter, to the last celery stalk, we all believed every last one of them was lying.

My friend Susan, a woman in her late fifties, was one such person. Susan has high blood pressure, and developed rheumatoid arthritis. She weighed two hundred and fifty pounds, and had been trying to lose weight for years. She tried every diet she could find, and stuck, or claimed she stuck, to each diet religiously. She asked me about every fad and every pill that came on the market – phen-phen, Merida, hypnosis, all approaches that were either unproven, ineffective over the long run, or would be proven to be dangerous. (One of the untoward effects of knowing a little physiology is knowing that there are no short cuts to weight loss. A person's weight is just the balance between what they take in, and what they burn. There are no shortcuts to simple math.) After Susan developed the rheumatoid arthritis, the need to lose weight became more acute – her weight was making the pain in her knees unbearable. Susan swore she was sticking to the 1500 calorie diet. I was doing my best to believe her – I had known her for years, and trusted her more than I trusted myself – but the old medical school teaching was always in the back of my mind. Susan must be a liar.

And that was when I got it. Susan was telling the truth. I was the liar.

I didn't know for sure how recommendations like the 2000 calorie diet were put together, but suddenly it struck me: the recommendation must come from the FDA, the federal Food and Drug Administration. I didn't know the food industry well, but I did know the drug industry – any practicing doctor does. They are the guys with the pens and lunches, the guys who are always inventing new diseases, so they can sell us all stuff. It's the drug industry that has every specialist of note on their payroll, and lots of primary care doctors too – they had tried to get me on the payroll once. Every new hot study that comes out has to be read incredibly carefully, because the influence of drug company money is everywhere, and the results are almost always biased, despite being published in the most respected peer reviewed journals. Every recommendation has to be viewed with caution, because the experts on the expert panels are also the folks on the take. Sometimes practicing medicine in the US feels more like dealing with a bunch of Columbian drug lords than it does like helping people think out how to feel well and function best, and get an equal shot at a decent life. American medicine is now so infiltrated, so corrupt, that every recommendation is suspect.

So if the 2000 calorie diet comes from the FDA, and the food part of the FDA is anything like the drug part, what are the chances that the 2000 calorie diet is accurate and unbiased? If the food profiteers are anything like the drug profiteers, and the real nutritional need for most american adults is 1200 calories, or even 1000 calories, doesn't that mean the food corporations stand to lose something like a third of their sales if people found out and stopped eating unnecessarily?

Could the reason that Susan couldn't lose weight on 1500 calories a day be that Susan only needs 1200 or 1000 calories a day, and all the authorities were lying, and I was lying with them? Isn't it more likely that Susan is telling the truth, than a bunch of for-profit companies with something to gain from one specific answer is telling the truth?

And isn't that what fasting tells us about nutritional needs? You don't really lose weight that quickly when you fast, because you never needed to eat much to begin with.

It turns out, on close inspection, that there is no 2000 calorie per day recommendation.

In fact there are no recommendations for caloric intake at all. The FDA doesn't make recommendations for caloric intake. We all just think it does. But there is still a culture of consumption that is pushing too many calories at the American people, and we, the nutritional and medical profession, have been total failures at telling people how little they really need.

Whoops. Time to change how we think about nutrition and eating, and time to understand that we have a food distribution system that is only about profit, and not about sustenance.

OK, How Many Calories Do American Earthlings Actually Need ?

No one knows.

Let's put it another way.

We need only as many calories as we burn. But we don't know how many calories we burn. We know we are eating more than we burn, however, because of the epidemic of obesity in the US, and because most of us are gaining a pound or two a year, and we tend to do that for years on end.

Let's put it still another way. We need only as many calories as we burn when the body is lean (with a body mass index of less than 20) because the heavier you are, the more calories you need to burn to move the extra weight around.

Let's put it one more way. Until a person is at lean body mass, that person needs fewer calories than she or he burns, because burning more than you eat is the only way to get to lean body mass, and lean body mass is the best place to be. (See the Chapter called Lean.)

But the tale gets more interesting. Remember the "recommended" 2000 calorie a day diet? It turns out that there is no 2000 calorie a day recommendation from the FDA or the United States Department of Agriculture, the nice people who brought you four food groups. There is no scientific body that makes a recommendation about daily caloric intake. Not one. The FDA, working with the Food and Nutrition Board of the Institute of Medicine of the National Academy of Sciences, carefully studied average caloric intake of Americans, and they then use that information to help figure out how much of the percent daily value of different nutrients and minerals eating a certain food represents.[11]

---

11 The FDA required nutritional information is often both helpful and confusing, despite years of effort by the nutrition and health professionals in and out of government to make it helpful, and in spite of their interactions with the food industry, who would just as soon make it confusing enough that their advertising can convince you to buy something for the wrong reason. The FDA wants you to understand what percent of something like the recommended daily allowance of each specific energy source, nutrient, or vitamin listed is supplied by eating the designated portion of the food product contained in the package on which the label is printed. The label always lists the percent of "daily value" supplied if you eat either a 2000 calories diet or a 2500 calorie diet. What's the "daily value'? The daily value is a number that lets you figure out what proportion of the amount of a nutrient someone (but not the FDA) thinks you should ingest in a day is in a labeled food product. HELP!! The percent daily value is not actually a recommendation, though it references something called the

Note that the percent daily value listed on the package of all nutrients is not a recommendation either. The 2000 calorie column, and the 2500 calorie column, are just ways of helping you understand what percent of the "usual" (which means recommended by someone else, not us, in FDA-speak) intake of a nutrient you'd get from a portion in the labeled package if you ate a 2000 calorie diet and 2500 calorie diet, respectively. (Don't worry if all this is confusing. No one else understands this either.) The package information only uses 2000 calorie and 2500 calorie a day diet respectively, because that's the estimated energy requirement of women and men respectively, an estimate made from calculations years ago, and the whole process turns on the assumption that calculations of estimated energy requirements are correct, and that people are only taking in as much food as they can burn, an assumption that is likely incorrect on both counts.

We know from fasting that you lose weight much more slowly than it feels like you should, even when you aren't eating at all, which means you probably don't need to take in that many calories after all. But how much is "not many calories?"

No one knows. No one, other than the folks who experimented with the very low protein diets in the late 1970s and early 1980s, has ever tested feeding diets containing different amounts of calories to lots of people to see what happens to their weight and bodies and overall health. This kind of clinical trial is impossible to do well, because you'd have to find a way to keep people from eating anything other than what is in the diet, and you'd have to control for different levels of activity, and for body size and shape, and, if possible, even for emotional stress and underlying illness – all things that can impact energy expenditure and caloric need.

The central problem really is that caloric need varies from person to person, and from time to time, so each person's caloric need is specific to that person's life at any one time, which is why it's so hard to study how many calories everyone needs, and give an answer that works for everyone.

You know your caloric intake is right for the life you are living when your weight doesn't change over time.

recommended daily intake, which itself is an updated term for the RDA -- recommended daily allowance. The recommended daily allowance actually is a recommendation, but a recommendation from the National Academy of Sciences, which is different from the FDA. (The best I can make out, it was too complex politically for the FDA to make a recommendation itself, because of " input" from the food industry, so it took cover by making up new language (percent daily value) and then "blaming" any recommendation on the National Academy of Science. Talk about pretzel logic. See how capitalism makes democracy interesting? And how everything about food and nutrition is influenced by the profit motive?

But what if you want to change the life you are living? What if you want to change your weight?

So what's an earthling to do?

How much should we eat?

We'll show you how to find out in the chapter called Fasting to Find Out, in the next section, called The Art of Not Eating.

It turns out the only way to answer these questions is to try The Zero Calorie Diet.

Calories Are Everywhere

This chapter is not really going to be about fasting.

It's about a corollary of the lesson we just learned from fasting – that we just weigh too much, because we are throwing too much food into our bodies. People don't lose weight that quickly from fasting, because they didn't need to eat much to begin with.

In our culture, calories are everywhere. The US produces about 3900 calories, per person per day.[12] That idea becomes meaningful once you start eating 1000 or 1200 calories a day. You just don't need to eat much food despite living a life surrounded by advertisements promoting food with too many calories.

A hot dog with a roll has 350 calories. That means if you eat only 3 hot dogs a day, and nothing else, you'll probably gain weight.

One cup of plain pasta: 182 calories. Not bad with dinner. But grazing leftovers from the refrigerator, when you picked your way through 3 cups, means you've eaten half of the total calories you can consume in a day without gaining weight.

Driving with my family, I asked my wife to hit the convenience store and pick me up a snack while I was pumping gas, to hold me over to a late dinner. She brought me back a handheld glazed pie, the kind that comes individually wrapped and costs about a dollar. I ate it first, and looked at the wrapper only later. 485 calories. If I had eaten a second one, that would have meant no more eating for the day.

One double stuffed Oreo cookie: 140 calories. That means if you eat seven double stuffed Oreo cookies in one day, you shouldn't eat anything else. Any open package of double stuffed Oreo cookies is as radioactive as enriched uranium, as toxic as mustard gas. Who can walk by an open package of double stuffed Oreos, and only eat one?

---

12 Center for Science in the Public Interest. http://www.cspinet.org/nutritionpolicy/food_advertising.html. 12/2/2008 11:22 AM

A Big Mac, with medium fries and a coke: 1182 calories. Not a disaster, as long as you don't eat anything else that day.

Now think, for a moment, about being surrounded by calories. Carefully walk yourself through your day. Most of us skip breakfast, or grab a cup of coffee as we roll out the door. But then there is a table somewhere - near the water cooler, in the back of the meeting room, or in the lunch room, on which sits the cranberry loaf someone brought in, or the box of cookies left by a vendor, or a container of chocolate. 300 calories before you know what hit you. You grab a lunch. Anything from a fast food joint is 500 to 600 calories, and might be a thousand, or even 1500 calories. 1500 Calories, and it's only lunch. You come home and throw dinner together. Someone taught you about three food groups once, so there is always a starch – and boom, 700 to 1000 calories. Then you snack in front of homework or TV (if you are in front of TV, there are the voices pushing you to go eat something about every 30 seconds) – white corn chips, 130 calories for each 9 chips – another 300 calories before you know it. So there went a typical day, and you swallowed somewhere between 1800 and 2600 calories – when you only needed 1000 to 1200.

Why do we eat so much? Because it's there. Why is it there? Because someone is making money from it being there.

There are other explanations for why we eat so much. One, most of us eat because we are anxious, and eating is a way to calm anxiety, a psychological release that goes back to childhood, and the way our mothers calmed our crying (which was mostly a way to tell those mothers we were hungry) by feeding us. It's worth thinking, for a moment, about why most of us are anxious, which takes us back to the craziness of our culture, a culture in which we all get to worry about money, about the stock market, about our fractured family relationships and friendships, worry about dread diseases, about work and conflicts at work, about national security – we all worry about everything, essentially all the time. It's also worth thinking, for a moment, about who profits when we worry, and remembering that those who profit are always those with something to sell – food, medicine, insurance, cigarettes, the need to have employees show up on time, or just advertising itself. (The people who bring you the news, which is always a source of anxiety, profit from you reading the news because they can bring you advertising, which is usually a way to make you worry about other things, so that you will buy things to stop worrying.)

We eat to give us an excuse to be together. How often is the meal at a restaurant with friends that good a meal?

We eat because satiation makes us feel good. Know the relaxed feeling after eating a large bowl of pasta?

We eat because we confuse thirst and hunger. Because the body is always losing fluid and sodium, and the brain depends on blood volume to work, there are frequent brain signals to drink, which we often confuse with hunger. (Remember, the body stores energy as glycogen and fat, so we rarely need to eat to insure we have enough moment to moment energy. It's the moment to moment variations in blood volume that drives fluid and food seeking behavior, not the need for energy.)

But we don't eat for nutrition. We don't eat for sustenance. We eat to eat.

There's a vicious cycle here. We have a culture that makes us anxious, and we live in material abundance, so we eat. We spend too much on eating, so we worry. We gain too much weight, because we are not eating for sustenance, and that makes us worry more – about health, and illness, and about weight itself. So we eat more.

Does that explain the invasion of Iraq? No. Does that explain Abu Ghraib or Guantanamo Bay or the stock market crash? Not directly. But aren't all these things – eating for the wrong reasons, invading countries for the wrong reasons, imprisoning people for the wrong reasons, using money for the wrong reasons, all part of the same cultural attitude, which might be, simply put, we do it because we can, not because we should?

We have met the enemy, and he is us.

And that is why we need to step away, and learn to fast.

The Zero Calorie Diet.

Reflection. Choice. Perspective.

Lean.

Why Do We Need So Few Calories?

Rolled up any car windows lately? Walked over to the TV to change the channel? Walked up five flights of stairs lately? Cut wood all day, or put up hay?

The demographic change in the US is overwhelming, and our calorie needs changed as where and how we live have changed.

In 1900, the US was 80 percent rural, and most of the population worked in agriculture. Now 80 percent or more of us live in cities or their suburbs, and less than 3 percent of the population farms, and those who farm often use machines to farm. Driving a big grain combine is farming, but it involves sitting behind a wheel in an air conditioned cab. Taking in hay with a harvester that makes huge round bales that we move from place to place with a tractor is farming, but its very different work from cutting hay with a scythe and lifting it onto a hay wagon with a pitchfork, which was how hay was brought in just 100 years ago. Similarly, running a huge mining machine with automated controls is mining, but it's very different work from digging into the face of a seam of coal with a pick, and lifting the coal by hand into a cart, which is how mining was done even 40 years ago. That shift has had a huge impact on our culture, true, but it also has had a huge impact on our energy consumption. Sitting at a desk all day, or talking on the telephone, or walking from room to room, or sitting behind the wheel of a vehicle, which is now what most of us do, just doesn't consume much energy.

Not too many years ago, kids walked to school. In 1969, about half of all school children walked, and 87 percent of kids living within a mile of school walked or biked.[13] By 2004, less than 13 percent of American children walked or biked to school.[14]

The FDA's use of 2000 and 2500 calorie a day diets as the standard to measure percent daily value – use that is a calculation, not a recommendation - comes from a report first issued in 1968. [15]

---

13 Centers for Disease Control. Barriers to children walking to or from school. September 30, 2005. 54 (38): 949-952.
14 Science Daily. http://www.sciencedaily.com/releases/2008/03/080326161643.htm. 12/2/2008 11:44 AM
15 National Research Council. Recommended dietary allowances. 7th ed. Food and Nutrition Board, Washington, DC: National Academy Press; 1968.

The report has been revised a few times, but the use of the 2000 and 2500 calories a day diets as the standard to estimate the proportions in the daily value hasn't changed.[16] [17] Even worse, the 2000 and 2500 calories a day diets were based on elegant, careful calculations - calculations of energy expenditure, corrected for gender, health, weight, race and a zillion other things, some of which are based on evidence reported in 1958, when people lived a very different life (in the 2005 report, most of the evidence is from the 1990s). The Institute of Medicine folks calculated how many calories a day people needed by studying how many calories a day they computed people used. Calculated!!! No one ever checked to see what happens when you feed a 2000 calorie a day diet to people in the real world, and certainly not to people living in the real world of 2008. These incredibly careful and precise calculations were reviewed and approved by a team of experts, but no one checked their work!!! [18]

The 2000 and 2500 calories a day diets weren't based on any direct experimental evidence. NO ONE HAS EVER TESTED the impact of feeding people 2000 calories a day over time!!!!!!! Well, almost no one. In practice, the nation has tested feeding people 2000 calories a day and more for the last 40 years, and we have ended up with an epidemic of obesity, which has befallen a nation of people, many of whom were doing what they thought the FDA was telling them to do.[19] So much for estimated energy requirements, and so much for calculation. Whoops. The pencil slipped.

NOW, think about the last time you rolled down a car window, or dialed a telephone instead of pushing buttons, or got up to change the channel on your TV, or pushed a lawn mower, or even raked a lawn with a rake (instead of blowing the leaves around with a contraption that makes way too much noise, and consumes way too much power.) We don't even have to push the keys on a typewriter. The keys on a computer are touch sensitive, and don't really even need muscle power.

We have become the victims of our own success. But the Amish are said to consume 3000-6000 calories a day, and few are overweight. They eat more because they burn more.

---

16 National Research Council. Recommended dietary allowances. 10th ed. Food and Nutrition Board, Washington, DC: National Academy Press; 1989.
17 Institute of Medicine. Dietary Reference Intakes for Energy, Carbohydrate, Fiber, Fat, Fatty Acids, Cholesterol, Protein, and Amino Acids (Macronutrients), Washington, DC: National Academy Press; 2005.
18 Yates A.   Which Dietary Reference Intake Is Best Suited to Serve as the Basis for Nutrition Labeling for Daily Values? J. Nutr. 136:2457-2462, October 2006
19   The FDA, in its defense, wasn't actually telling people to do anything. It was just describing what most people do, trying to get to recommended intake of nutrients, not calories, made by others

They walk 7 to 9 miles a day, and do physical work at least 10 to 12 hours a week.[20]   The rest of us are lucky if we walk a tenth of a mile a day, and do physical work for a few minutes a day. We burn way less, and so we need to eat way less. Way less. So we can weigh less.

But wait – it gets worse. The average American spends 6 hours a day watching video-based entertainment, 4 hours of which is spent watching television.[21] That's 4 to 6 hours a day, bathed in commercial messages encouraging people to eat more. But it's worse still. There is evidence, from studies of children, that when you watch television, your resting energy expenditure drops to less than when you are laying down, and presumably, less than when you are sleeping.[22]   Since metabolic activity at rest is mostly a function of brain activity, it looks like the brain stops working when you watch TV (something parents have been telling children for years!). It's as if your brain gets taken over by the television producers, and the brain lets the television process do its work for it, replacing obsessing, cogitating, thinking and dreaming – with just watching, as if your brain was hibernating, stuck in neutral, the engine on but just barely turning over.

One interesting observation is that no one ever voted to eliminate the window cranks from car doors, just like no one ever voted to get rid of dial telephones, just like no one ever voted to put in telephones to replace walking down the street to talk to family or friends, and no one ever voted on watching 6 hours of television a day. It happened, as if by itself, all driven by the desire of some of us to make a buck.

Here's the second major explanation, then, of why people don't lose weight that quickly when they fast, and, parenthetically, why it's hard to lose weight at all. We don't do much. We don't burn the food we eat, and we are actually pretty efficient, so we can run on very little fuel when there isn't much exercise. With fasting, the body actually gets more efficient – the body limits activity and uses energy exceptionally well. And by not exercising, we are actually imitating the response of the body to fasting itself - from a physiologic point of view, the body might call our absence of exertion plenty in the midst of starvation. That is, we have plenty of fuel, but we aren't using it. And our bodies, along with our culture and our souls, are showing the strain of doing too little physical work, just as we are doing too much eating, all for no real purpose other than

---

20 Roberts, W. The Amish, body weight, and exercise.The American Journal of Cardiology, Volume 94, Issue 9, Pages 1221-1221.

21 http://www.tvweek.com/news/2008/06/web_video_consumption_seen_hit.php. 12/3/2008 8:25 AM

22 Klesges RC, Shelton ML, Klesges LM. Effects of television on metabolic rate: potential implications for childhood obesity. Pediatrics. 1993 Feb;91(2):281-6.

someone else's profit.

The change in human activity has occurred gradually, almost evolutionarily. Pieces of ourselves – the pieces connected to working hard together, farming or hunting; the pieces connected to walking down the street to check on each other, the pieces connected to not having that much to eat, but eating together, have also been lost, swept away without our even noticing their disappearance.

Fasting tells us why it's hard to lose weight quickly. It also tells us something about who we've become, whether or not we want to be the people we are.

No one chose the life or culture we have. Few of us chose to invade Iraq. Fewer of us actively and passionately resisted that invasion.

The Zero Calorie Diet.

Reflection. Memory. Perspective. Thinking about the choices we made - and the choices we didn't make, or don't even notice we made, or let be made for us while we were out sea kayaking, or watching TV.

Why Stomach Stapling Works

Bariatric surgery drives me crazy. Bariatric surgery, which most people call stomach stapling, helps people lose weight. There are actually a couple of different operations that surgeons use, some of which work better than others. Like any major surgery, there are potential complications; and the surgery costs thousands – even tens of thousands – of dollars….. but it works. People who have it really do lose weight – often hundreds of pounds, and their diabetes goes away, their blood pressure returns to normal, their heart disease risk returns to normal, they look more attractive, feel better about themselves, and get to live happily every after.

So why does it drive me crazy?

Bariatric surgery drives me crazy because it represents a culture of excess, a culture where we have lost all of our self-control, a culture run by marketing, and marketeers. There is nothing bariatric surgery does that people can't do for themselves. Only we've convinced the people who have the surgery that they "can't" not eat.

Say what?

Bariatric surgery is just a mechanical way of inducing a fast. There is no magic here. Bariatric surgery is the nutritional equivalent of a chastity belt. It's an admission that some of us are incapable of resisting the lure of advertising and cheap calories. It's giving in, a way of admitting that we do not control our own choices.

There is nothing that you get from bariatric surgery that you don't get from simply limiting your own intake to 600 or 1000 calories a day.

Interestingly, there is no increase in reported sudden deaths in people who undergo bariatric surgery. Why? No one knows. No reported deaths doesn't mean cardiac sudden death doesn't occur. It just means no one has reported an increased incidence of sudden death among people who have had their stomachs stapled. It's not clear why this experience is different from the experience of low calorie protein sparing fasts in the late seventies. It could be that the caloric intake after bariatric surgery, about twice that of the protein sparing fasts, is enough to prevent wasting of what's called the cardiac skeleton, the tissue that controls heart rate and rhythm, and which was thought to be the problem with the protein sparing fasts. It could be that people exercise after bariatric surgery, which was usually not the case with protein sparing fasts, and exercise preserves the cardiac skeleton. It could be that we are much better at watching out for and reducing high cholesterol now, so that the underlying risk of heart disease and sudden death is less. It could be that protein sparing fasts were used only for people who were truly massively obese, and bariatric surgery is used for people who do not weigh as much, important because there are disturbances of the heart's rhythm which are reported as weight increases. But the difference is striking, and we should pay attention to it over time, to see if it is a real difference, or if, in the course of time, the problem of sudden death associated with severe fasting reasserts itself.

No one makes people eat. No one made us invade Iraq. Sometimes, it makes sense to stop and think about who we are, what we really need, and what we can do without.

The Great Low Fat Low Cholesterol Scam

Low cholesterol is not low calorie. Stamp out greed.

One of the great things about The Zero Calorie Diet is that you get to ignore what's supposed to be good for you and what's supposed to be bad for you, because you don't eat anything. Indeed, the obsession with the nutritional value of food, which Michael Pollan and others call nutritionism, probably contributes to the uniquely American post-industrial, and very deep, anxieties, which themselves often lead to obsessive eating.[23]

But if you are eating, one of the traps you will need to deal with is the low cholesterol, low fat diet trap, which is similar in many ways to the low or no carbohydrate trap, the high protein diet trap, the caveman diet trap, the grapefruit diet trap, the organic food trap, the whole wheat diet trap, and every other dietary scam that has ever come down the pike.

Fasting teaches you that diets don't matter, because you don't lose weight that quickly even if you eat nothing.

I'll say it again. Weight depends only on the difference between what you take in and what you burn. Measured in calories. Only the caloric content matters for weight. Nothing else has any meaning for weight. The stripe, color, character, name, genealogy, family history, social conditions, race, place of origin of the food you eat - none of it matters, from the perspective of maintaining a healthy weight, and avoiding the diabetes, heart disease, stroke and cancers we cause by being too fat. From the perspective of maintaining a healthy weight, the only thing that matters is burning what you take in, and taking in no more than you need, in calories. (There, I said it every way I can think of. Forgive me for being redundant, but people just don't seem to get this, and there are a zillion people with something to sell who are trying to convince you that the obvious just ain't true. They are wrong. It's all just addition and subtraction.)

Now, that doesn't mean diet isn't important for other things beside weight, and that's where the confusion comes. Diet is important for lots of other things. But most people focus on the relationship between diet and weight, sometimes for

23 Pollan, Michael. In Defense of Food –an eater's manifesto. (New York: The Penguin Press, 2008)

health, but more often because advertisers are also trying to sell everyone on the importance of "having" a perfect looking body, so people are motivated to use diet to change their weight, and people with something to sell take advantage of that motivation.

So, let's think for a moment about the low cholesterol, low fat diet scam. First principle. Eating a low fat diet or low cholesterol diet has nothing to do with losing or maintain weight. The "low-fat" in "low-fat diet" means only that you are taking in a diet lower than usual in fats you ingest. It doesn't mean the diet will make you less fat. This may seem obvious when stated, but it took me, despite years of medical training, years to get it right – the words are seductive and confusing.

Low fat and low cholesterol diets are there to help you lower your cholesterol, and thereby reduce your risk of heart disease. A part of that risk comes from cholesterol when cholesterol is high, and lowering cholesterol, independently from lowering weight, reduces the risk of heart disease in populations of people who are at greater risk because their cholesterol is high.

Sound simple? It isn't. The words and ideas lie. First thing you have to know: about half of the people who have heart disease have normal cholesterol, so lowering your cholesterol may not protect you from heart disease. Second thing you have to know: not everyone who eats a diet low in cholesterol or fat is successful in lowering their cholesterol. Third thing you have to know: lots of people with high cholesterol live to 100 and never get heart disease – the association between low cholesterol and less heart disease is a population effect, which may or may not impact the health of individuals. Say what?

A population effect. If we can lower the cholesterol of 100 people with established heart disease, who have a risk of about 30 in 100 of developing new heart disease over 10 years, only 21 to 24 of those people, instead of 30, will develop new heart disease, which sounds like a small effect although it is a good thing, but there's a problem: we don't know who among the 100 people at higher risk will benefit from lowering their cholesterol. So while lowering your cholesterol with diet or medication lowers the likelihood that 100 people like you will develop new heart disease, we don't know whether or not it will help *you* avoid heart disease.

But wait, it gets worse yet. The strongest evidence that lowering cholesterol will help a few people avoid heart disease is for people with heart disease already. The evidence supporting the notion that lowering cholesterol in asymptomatic people is still pretty weak, the effect is small, and that effect is a population effect, not an individual outcome effect.

So what is the right choice? Low fat, low cholesterol – or throw caution to the wind?

Despite everything I just said, I still think it makes sense to eat a calorie conscious diet lower in fats, but it doesn't make sense to drive yourself crazy doing it, and the calorie conscious part is probably more important than the low fat part, everything else being equal. Why? The drift of all the evidence is that lower cholesterol is probably better for you. There's lots of additional evidence suggesting being lean, having little body fat, and getting plenty of exercise, is associated with longevity. I eat little meat – but some, stay away from fried foods, and keep my diet to 1000-1200 calories a day, which is plenty for someone who works outside hauling wood, or gardening 1-2 hours a day.

Should someone with high cholesterol take medicine? It depends on how high their cholesterol is, what the LDL and HDL is, what the ratio between cholesterol and HDL is, and, most importantly, on their family history. Someone with high cholesterol and a close family history of early heart disease probably should think about taking cholesterol lowering medicine, if they can't lower their cholesterol by diet and exercise, which they should try first.

What about all the other diets out there? All the other diets out there have to be considered individually, because they are meant, like the low fat diet, to achieve different things. The only way to reduce or maintain weight is to keep your intake less or equal to what you burn in calories. Most diets are tricks to help you do that, but the ones that aim at weight maintenance all do it the same way – they help you limit calories.

So Weight Watchers, the caveman diet, high and low protein diets, the grapefruit and watermelon diets, the South Beach diet are all different versions of the same thing. They get people to focus on calories, using mostly behavioral, or quasi pharmacological tricks, to help reduce calories by distracting you or helping you to manage what you perceive to be hunger, and is mostly thirst, and eating behaviors caused by anxiety. But if they work, they work only to the extent to which they get you to limit your caloric intake, or increase your exercise.

Whole foods or natural foods have a different purpose. They are there to reduce your exposure to chemicals and additives which may themselves be harmful. They may help you to live longer or feel better, but they have nothing to do with

maintaining weight. It's possible to gain weight by eating only organic broccoli, if you (can bear to) eat 5000 calories of broccoli a day, just like its possible
to lose weight if you eat only McDonald's French fries, as long as you only eat
500 calories worth in a day, and nothing else.

Each style of eating has a purpose. The analysis of nutritional claims always
brings us back to the same place. We don't need to eat much, and simple and
cheap is as good as or better than fancy, wrapped, and advertised. When someone makes a claim for something, it's because they are trying to sell you something, not because they are trying to improve your health.

Here's what we learn from The Zero Calorie Diet about other diets of all sorts.
Everything connected to food in our culture, even eating less, is about someone
trying to sell you something.

Stamp out greed.

Part IV - The Art Of Not Eating

The Art Of Not Eating

Figuring out that we eat way more calories than we need, and why we do that, was the easy part. Now comes the hard part. How to eat less. How to balance thirst, which we often confuse with hunger, contain the anxiety we get from living in a society that seems out of control, resist food-like products full of calories that are everywhere, and stare down the barrage of messages from all media, saying, individually and in chorus, eat more. And oh, add physical work to a busy day. Doing physical work isn't the same as not eating, but it carries many of the same benefits, in terms of avoiding or postponing heart disease, diabetes, stroke, and cancer, that staying lean does, and it helps you stay lean, as long as you don't eat too much after working.

One promise. I'm not going to try to sell you anything, other than this book. Not now, not ever. Most ways of not eating are put forth by someone trying to profit out of them, which has its own set of problems, as we create a world of mistrust, which comes from a world in which people are always trying to put something over on each other, in order to create profit for themselves. These ideas are just ideas that have worked for me and people who have been my patients. It's fine with me if you read this book standing between the aisles of a bookstore. Or better, borrow it from a library. If every library in the US buys it, I'll do fine – the idea isn't to make a big fortuna writing this. The idea is to see us all at a place where we can hang out without worrying, and watch our children grow up without feeling like we need to invade small foreign countries chasing their oil, where we eat less because that's all we need, and fasting as penitence isn't often necessary.

Drink Deep And Often

The easiest way to avoid eating is to drink all day long – but drink something without calories, since lots of drinks – soda, juice, beer or anything with alcohol, are chock full of calories. How chock full? Most sodas and juices contain 100-120 calories per 8 ounce glass. Since I'm about to tell you to drink at least 3 quarts, or 12 to 15 different 8 ounce glasses of water a day, that would be 800 to 1400 calories per day, which is fine, in terms of taking in as many calories as you need, as long as you eat nothing else. (Not really fine – if you drank only juice or soda, you might take in enough calories, but you'd miss lots of other nutrients which you need. Drink, but don't only drink, unless you are fasting).

Why drink? Remember, you lose 1 percent of your total body fluid volume every day by breathing and in sweat, urine, and stool. You notice changes in your performance once you lose 2 percent of your total body fluid volume. But even before the loss of fluid impacts your performance, your body senses the loss (by sensing a change in the cells of the hypothalamus, in the brain) and sends a message, which you perceive as thirst, to the brain. Doctors believe people confuse hunger and thirst, so these little changes in blood volume and concentration that occur all day long trigger the eating that is better to avoid.

It turns out the confusion of hunger and thirst may not be confusion after all. If you drink only water, you don't replace the sodium which you are also losing all the time, and the fluid you drink won't keep your blood volume expanded enough to keep bringing blood to the brain. So because you "confuse" hunger and thirst, and eat, you take in enough sodium to keep your blood volume up. The only problem is what you eat. When we lived in the days of nuts and berries, and nibbled all the time, you'd get enough sodium to support your blood volume, you'd get lots of fiber, but you wouldn't get many calories. But living in the days of Oreos, Twinkies, and Big Macs, nibbling causes you to ingest lots of calories, makes you fat, and causes all the Western diet diseases – diabetes, high blood pressure, heart disease, stroke, and cancer. Same nibbling, different time. Relative rates.

(So I need to be clear for a moment - the hypothalamus is a bit of neuroendocrine tissue and doesn't think on its own, so the hypothalamus doesn't "confuse" hunger and thirst. We confuse hunger and thirst, because we are confused about how the body works. Thirst triggers the hunger needed to cause you to replace the sodium you are always losing, so the body can both have adequate fluid and maintain enough blood volume to bring blood to the brain. The body is actually pretty smart, for being just a body. Doctors, on the other hand, who think the body does only what they think it does, and for only the reasons they know about...well, maybe doctors ought to fast more.)

How much fluid do you lose every day? A well hydrated person puts out about 1.5 liters of urine, and loses 1 liter by breathing and in sweat, urine, and stool, for a total of 2.5 liters. You lose more if you're anxious, doing hard physical work or exercise (or anything else that makes you sweat), or if it's a hot day.

Losing 3 liters a day without replacing any of that fluid is the medical definition of shock! (The medical definition of shock is losing more than 20 percent of your extra-cellular fluid, most of which is in your circulatory system. The extra-cellular volume is 12-14 liters. Twenty percent of 14 liters is 2.8 liters.)

So the most time sensitive nutrients are fluid and sodium, because you are losing them all the time, and because the body doesn't store them well. You have a 1 day reserve of fluid. You have a 1-2 day reserve of sodium (which is actually stored in other places besides fluid, but not stored that well). Most Americans have a 3 to 12 month reserve of energy. Which means if you start to eat less, you should think about replacing the fluid and the sodium, but essentially forget about replacing calories, until you are at your lean weight, which is scathingly low. (I'm 5'10, and weigh 185, down from 225. I weighed 160 in high school. My lean weight is 130-140. I could go 4 to 6 more months without eating before worrying about calories.) You can find your lean weight by figuring out what you would need to weigh for your gender, height, and build at a body mass index of 20, using the body mass index chart in the appendix.

How much should you drink? Eight to fifteen 8 ounce glasses of water a day. Most authorities say eight 8 ounces glasses. Our friends at the Food and Nutrition Board of the Institute of Medicine think the right amount is 91 ounces – twelve 8 ounces glasses of water for women and twelve to fifteen 8 ounce glasses for men, and I think they are basically correct, but some authorities think that's way too much, and you should only drink when you are thirsty.[24][25]

24 Institute of Medicine. Daily Reference Guides: Water, Potassium, Sodium, Chloride and Sulfate. National Academies Press, 2004.
25 Negoianu D. Goldfarb S. Just add water. J Am Soc Nephrol 2008; Jun 19(6):1041-3.

How do you know whether or not you are drinking enough fluid? By how much you pee, and how wet your mouth is. It's astoundingly simple. If you are urinating a decent amount every 4 to 6 hours, and your mouth is moist, you are drinking enough. If you are urinating only once in 12 hours, and your mouth is dry, you aren't drinking enough. This is a simple measure that works everywhere, which is important, because your fluid needs change with outside temperature and exercise. So if you are working outside, and sweating up a storm, and you notice your mouth is dry, and that you haven't urinated in 8 hours, but you are drinking a bottle every few hours, stop! And drink more. Although your intake of fluid is there, it's just not enough. Pay attention, and make sure you drink enough to support your needs and losses, particularly when you are fasting, and particularly after you've reduced your intake of calories.

The reason I think The Institute of Medicine's suggestion that you need 12 to 15 eight ounce glasses of water a day is correct is because of the moment to moment fluctuation in fluid volume, and how that fluctuation can impact hunger, and how you feel. You need to understand that there is no hard evidence whatsoever that drinking more is associated with less hunger, weight loss, or a person's ability to sustain a long fast. But replacing your fluid losses quickly is likely to have those effects, and has few risks. (There are risks to way over-replacing fluid losses – something called water intoxication, but the Institute of Medicine's recommendations are only aimed at replacing likely daily losses, and not overdoing it.) There are individual variations in fluid needs, of course, but because for most of us excess water is so easy to eliminate, overshooting slightly is just no big deal, and having plenty of fluid in your system, what might be called a full tank, has lots of potential benefits, and the benefits far outnumber the tiny potential risks.

How Much (Or How Little)?

*Using The Zero Calorie Diet To Answer
One Of Life's Persistent Questions*

Figuring out how much to drink is easy. Your fluid needs are pretty standard, and don't vary much from person to person. Everyone needs to drink at least 2.5 liters a day – more if you are in hot weather, or working hard enough to sweat.

Figuring out how much, or little, to eat is more complicated.

It turns out that the only way to find out how much to eat is to fast. There are a bunch of formulas you could use (see appendix) that let you calculate what your caloric need might be – but they are formulas, estimates, derived from the study of other people from another time, and because they are calculations, they don't tell you what YOU use and need. If you want to know what you need and what you use, you'll need to fast.

Remember how the caloric need of each person varies from person to person? Remember that no scientific body has a recommendation for how many calories a day you should eat?

Here's how to use a fast to find out how many calories you burn.

First, buy a decent but inexpensive digital bathroom scale. The decent ones do weight in 0.2 pound increments, and let you display your weight in either the English or Metric scale. They run off lithium batteries, and cost $20-30 dollars. (I bought one in the local discount store for $20.)

Choose a good day to start a three day fast. A good day to start a fast is when you aren't stressed, and don't have three impossibly heavily loaded work days in front of you, don't need to travel, and aren't going to run a marathon or have some other physically strenuous days planned. The time when your body switches from burning stored carbohydrate to burning fat is unpredictable, and there are often a few hours of tiredness that occur after your carbohydrate stores have run down, but before your body has converted to burning fat. That conversion happens anywhere between 12 and 36 hours of fasting, but it makes your performance during the fast, which is generally pretty normal, somewhat unpredictable for a few hours,

(Check with your doctor first, to make sure nothing about your health prevents you from a 3 day food but not fluid fast. Most doctors will think you are nuts – not because there is any health risk, but because fasting is not something doctors are programmed to think about. When you are a hammer, you think the world is a nail. Ignore the pejorative comments about being a health nut. Doctors, who actually believe in the medications they prescribe, are just as much health nuts as you are. Just make sure there is nothing in your medical history that would make fasting dangerous. Diabetics on medication, and people taking long term medications, probably shouldn't do a 3 day fast - not that there is anything dangerous about the fast per se – but because many medications rely on a regular food and fluid intake to keep a stable concentration of the medication in the blood and tissues.)

On awakening the morning you are going to start the fast, weigh yourself three times, naked, after you've used the toilet. If two of the weights are the same, use that number. If the weights are all a little different, but within 8 tenths of a pound, add them and divide by three, and use that number. If the weights are more than a pound different, replace the battery in the scale, or get a new scale. $30 scales aren't perfect, but most of the time they'll do, and don't worry if the weight they show is different from what you weigh in the doctor's office. The scale doesn't have to be perfectly accurate. The scale just has to be consistent enough so that the difference in your weight before and after fasting is close enough to accurate to let you calculate how many calories you burn a day accurately. (Use this procedure of taking three weights every time you weigh yourself for this exercise.)

Write down the time and date, the fact that you weighed yourself naked after using the toilet, and the weight, down to the "tenths" place.

Then don't eat anything but 1 to 2 cups of bouillon (the kind you make from powder or foil wrapped cubes) once or twice a day for three days. How much to drink depends on how much sodium is in each cup. You want no more than 1.5 to 2 grams of sodium. Drink plenty of clear liquids, at least 12 glasses of water or clear liquid a day. (Not juice though, because juice has lots of calories.) That combination gives you 2 grams of sodium, 3 liters of water, and only 40 calories a day. Enough to support your blood volume and get the blood flowing to the brain, and a countable intake of calories that is also so small that you will burn existing body stores, so we can measure how much you've needed to burn simply by weighing you.

If you start to feel badly, go ahead and eat – this fast isn't that important, though the information it produces is interesting.

Keep doing what you always do. The same amount of exercise. The same amount of work. The same amount of laughter. The same amount of worry. The same amount of stress. The same amount of play. The same amount of TV, if you must (but believe me, there is nothing worth watching). The same amount of computer time. The same amount of sex. Roughly the same amount of everything, since everyone's day varies. (The reason for doing 3 days is that method captures more day to day variation. The longer the fast, the more accurate the information, but few of us are ready for more than a three day fast.)

On the morning of the fourth day, just after you get out of bed (after three days of no solid food) weigh yourself again, naked, after you've used the toilet.

Write down the weight. Then have a snack if you want one.

Subtract the fourth day's weight from the first day's weight.

Multiply that result by 3500 (the number of calories per pound of fat).

Subtract 120 (the number of calories you got from the bouillon.)

Divide by 3.

The number you have is the maximum number of the calories per day you are consuming.

Now take the number you multiplied by 3500, and multiply it by 1555 instead. That's the number of calories per pound of protein and carbohydrate.

Subtract 120 (again, the number of calories you got from the bouillon.)

Divide that by three.

That number is the minimum number of calories per day you are consuming.

Take the maximum number and the minimum number, add them together, and divide by 2. That gives you a sense of your actual daily caloric requirement.

The difference between the minimum and maximum number of calories represents the energy source of the calories you are burning, which isn't possible to measure simply in a real person, remembering that fat has 9 calories per gram or about 3500 calories per pound, and protein and carbohydrate have 4 calories per gram, or about 1555 per pound. That is, since it's not possible to know how much fat you are burning at any one time early in a fast, and how much stored carbohydrate or protein from muscle breakdown you are burning early in the fast, we compute the caloric consumption from both sources, to get a feel for the real number, because the body gradually transitions from using carbohydrate to using fat as an energy source over about 2 weeks.

Let's do a sample calculation.

Say I weigh 185.4 on the first day and 184.2 on the fourth day. The difference is 1.2 pounds. 1.2 times 3500 equals 4200. 4200 minus 120 equals 4080. 4080 divided by 3 equals 1360.

Now repeat the calculation. 1.2 times 1555 equals 1866. 1866 minus 120 equals 1746. 1746 divided by 3 equals 582.

So the least number of calories I am burning a day is 582, and the most is 1360 calories. A reasonable rule of thumb is just to average the two values, to get a rough estimate of the truth. 582 plus 1360 is 1942, divided by 2 is 971. That's 971 calories a day – your personal calorie consumption, measured by you, for you, in your own life.

Check your own number. I'll bet it's 1000-1400 calories a day, unless you are a workout king or queen. If you do an hour of strenuous, huffing and puffing kind of exercise, the number will likely come out 1400-1800 calories a day.

If you put together three pieces of critical information – how few calories you really need in a day, how many calories there are – in everything you eat – and how far you really are from your lean weight, you'll be able to not eat when eating isn't necessary.

Now you know how much you can eat, and maintain your weight and health, in your own life.

All you have to do is drop down from what you are now eating, to what you can

58

eat, and remember to not eat.

Not so hard, but there is an art to not eating, which, because of the way the body manages fluid and sodium, doesn't come naturally to any of us. Even when you are not eating by just drinking, it's still tricky to remember not to eat, and to drink instead, when food products are everywhere, and there is always food product propaganda in the air.

Still, think back on The Zero Calorie Diet, when you are tempted to eat unnecessarily and just follow the directions you've learned. When you get right down to it, easy to follow directions are right on the box.

The Song Of Salt, Redux

Salt, **sodium** chloride, is the food that we most commonly eat to get sodium, an element that is important in maintaining blood volume, the size and shape of cells, and the transmission of electrical impulses in the body. Most of the sodium in the body is in the body's fluids. We lose sodium all the time in urine, sweat and feces, and don't store sodium that well – you only have enough sodium to keep your sodium level stable for a day or so unless you ingest more sodium, something we are doing constantly. There is sodium in almost all foods, with processed or preserved foods being loaded with sodium (and calories). Only a few foods have lots of sodium without being loaded with calories. Sodium is necessary to maintain your blood volume and bring blood to the brain. Fluid alone doesn't maintain blood volume. Because of the way the kidneys work, if you have enough fluid, and not enough sodium, your kidneys will dump the fluid anyway. It's fluid and sodium together that are necessary to keep the concentration of sodium in the blood what it should be, and bring blood to the brain.

Adding sodium to your diet when you reduce your intake is the other part of not eating as much. But please remember. I am not advocating using extra sodium. I am advocating adding salt to bring your sodium intake back to what it was before you reduced your caloric intake, which also reduced your salt intake, something most people don't realize they are doing when they reduce the calories they are eating. Supplement salt for a week or two, until your kidneys catch up to the change in salt intake by doing a better job of hanging on to the sodium in your body. Then gradually stop supplementing salt.

Don't increase your total sodium, and don't supplement sodium for very long. The extra sodium is a short term measure, designed to help you tolerate the changes in blood volume that accompany eating less in the short term.

Here's what happens when you reduce your caloric intake. Your sodium intake falls with your caloric intake, but your kidneys keep letting sodium flow out of the body, because it takes time for the kidneys to adjust to the reduced sodium. The loss of sodium means your blood becomes more concentrated, and your blood volume shrinks, which means less blood to the brain in the short term. Once your blood becomes more concentrated, and your blood volume shrinks, your kidneys start to hold on to sodium instead of letting so much out in the urine, but that change takes time – about 2 weeks. (When your blood becomes concentrated and the blood volume shrinks you also become thirsty and hungry together, as the body tries to correct the low blood volume by getting you to eat and drink more.) It's during those two weeks that the supplementation of sodium is so helpful, because it prevents hunger and thirst, and keeps you from eating more.

There's plenty of evidence that about one third of people with high blood pressure benefit from salt restriction, and lots of people think that too much salt over time has some of the adverse health consequences of the western diet – here, high blood pressure, heart disease and stroke. But it's not that hard to sort out how to balance the health benefits from reducing weight with the health benefits of reducing sodium, which have been estimated to save 150,000 lives a year if the average consumption of sodium could be reduced by 50 percent.[26] Estimates of the excess deaths per year from obesity have ranged all over the map – from about 120,000 to 400,000 or more, and don't take into account the illnesses and costs associated with obesity associated diabetes and heart disease.[27] So there are benefits from reducing weight and benefits from reducing sodium.

How do you reduce both weight and sodium intake? Do one at a time. Accept staying at your sodium level for a period of time, drop your food intake, then drop your weight, then bring your sodium intake down as your total calorie intake falls, but after the body gets used to the reduced sodium intake that comes with reducing calories.

Say what?

Start slowly. First reduce your calorie intake, but keep your sodium intake the same, so you don't get thirsty and hungry together – so you can keep your calorie intake lower over time, which will reduce your weight.

Then gradually, over 2 weeks, stop taking the extra salt, as your body becomes used to the reduced amount of salt you are taking in, and uses the sodium in the salt effectively, maintaining your blood volume and blood concentration on a reduced intake of both calories and sodium.

26 Havas S, Roccella EJ, Lenfant C. Reducing the public health burden from elevated blood pressure levels in the United States by lowering intake of dietary sodium. Am J Public Health 2004;94:19–22

27 Flegal KM, Graubard BI, Williamson DF, Gail MH. Excess deaths associated with underweight, overweight, and obesity. JAMA. 2005 Apr 20;293(15):1861-7

The recommended daily salt intake is 3.8 grams, of which 1.5 grams is sodium.[28] The recommended sodium intake is 1.5 to 2.3 grams.[29] Diet recall studies suggest that the average sodium intake is 3375 milligrams a day, though some observers think it is higher.[30] (The numbers get confusing here because of the difference between salt and sodium. Salt is *sodium chloride* - one gram of *salt* contains 387 milligrams of sodium; one teaspoon of salt contains 6200 milligrams of salt and 2400 milligrams of sodium.)

No reasonable human being should sit around and count the milligrams of salt or sodium he or she takes in a day. So how do you manage your salt intake?

It's pretty simple. Know about a couple of high salt, low calorie foods, and guesstimate, being ready to overshoot a little - but just a little, and not for long.

For example, bouillon ranges from 500 milligrams to 1400 milligrams of sodium in each cup. If you've cut your calorie intake from 2000 calories a day to 1200 calories a day, your sodium intake dropped by about a third, or from approximately 3.5 grams a day, to about 2.0 grams a day, leaving you about 1.5 grams a day to make up. So you can drink 3 cups of the 500 milligram of lower sodium bouillon, or 1 to 2 cups of the 1300 milligram of higher sodium bouillon, to make up the difference. If you are fasting, your sodium intake goes to zero, so you need 3.5 grams of sodium a day, at least in the short term - or seven cups of the lower sodium bouillon, or about 3 cups of the higher sodium bouillon, to make up the difference.

Pickles each contain about 250 milligrams of sodium, and about 5 calories. So you could eat 5 or 6 pickles a day to make up the sodium difference if you reduce your food intake by one third, without getting lots of calories. (You probably don't want to use pickles if you are fasting and mean not to eat.)

The point is to think about sodium as you reduce your calorie intake, so you can reduce your caloric intake successfully. It doesn't help to understand the value of reducing your intake, unless you can eat less now and keep eating less for the rest of your life. Diets are nice. Eating less forever is a change in how you think, who you are, and how we are together, as we together begin to understand how to control our addiction to excess, and learn to think about who benefits when we get it wrong.

28 Institute of Medicine. Daily reference intakes: Water, Potassium, Sodium, Chloride and Sulfate. National Academies Press, 2004.
29 Institute of Medicine. Dietary reference intakes: water, potassium, sodium, chloride, and sulfate. Washington, DC: National Academies Press, 2004.
30 http://www.cdc.gov/nchs/data/nhanes/databriefs/calories.pdf

Shoot The Refrigerator

About a year ago, our refrigerator died, and, when we couldn't find a new one that "fit" where the old one had been, I decided we didn't need to replace it, and we lived without a refrigerator for a year.

When we moved to a house in the country 15 years ago, the house came with an expensive, trendy, built-in refrigerator, installed by the previous owners as they tried to give a simple, drafty, antique colonial built in the 1730s, country chic.

Before long, the refrigerator, built more for style than quality, started to break down.

For the first few years of its breaking down, we tried to fix it.

Each year we'd fix it, and spent more each year than a new store-bought refrigerator cost.

And then last year we gave up, and had the darn thing hauled away. It had lived in an odd shaped space, and there really was no store-bought refrigerator that fit in the space, so we struggled for a while, trying to figure out what to do.

And that was when it struck me.

Part of our problem with weight and eating is that we all have these great big refrigerators that we really don't need. I looked inside ours. Most of what is there is leftovers. Most of the way we use leftovers is for grazing. One of us gets hungry, goes to the refrigerator, and then stands there opening containers, one after the next, surfing the leftovers.

(It turns out this kind of grazing is a common way people eat too many calories. It's hard to know how much you are eating, when you are standing at the refrigerator, nibbling through one container, and then the next. That's why nutritionists often urge people to put food on a plate when they are eating, and sit down with others, so you can actually think about what you are eating, remembering that is usually triggered by anxiety or a TV commercial, not hunger. Remember, most of us carry 3 to 6 months of energy stores. We almost never "need' to eat. We only barely need to eat meals, which are times to be with the people you love and not times to pile in the calories - and certainly don't "need" to eat *between* meals.)

I suddenly realized that the best way to keep from having too many leftovers is not to cook too much. Then I realized that a better way to keep from rummaging through the refrigerator, looking for leftovers, is just not to have a refrigerator to rummage through. Having no refrigerator would keep us from mindless eating, keep us from mindless shopping, and save electricity and fossil fuel, since the refrigerator is the household appliance that consumes the most electricity.

Sounds pretty simple. It was. Having no refrigerator was better then simple. It worked, and it had lots of unexpected benefits. Having no refrigerator just took a little while to get used to.

Having no refrigerator means you have to shop every few days – but that's a good thing, because everything you eat is fresh, not frozen. Having no refrigerator means you are much more likely to stop at a farm stand or farmer's market, which is good for the local economy, as you are spending money on local people's work, and not on fossil fuels which allow us to take advantage of low paid workers halfway across the hemisphere. Having no refrigerator means you occasionally spend time talking to the people who staff the farm stands or farmer's markets, who are, after all, your neighbors. Having no refrigerator means you think about how much you are going to eat at each meal, and buy just what you need, so there is less waste, no leftovers, and less expense.

True, after a while, we started using a little dorm refrigerator, which we had been storing in the basement for years, so we could comfortably keep eggs, milk and butter. True, we have a chest freezer out on a porch, where we store meat and the few frozen foods we use. But you can't graze a chest freezer, and the freezer doesn't use much energy.

So why do we all have these big, white behemoths that drink energy, take up space, and make us all fat?

After a refrigerator free year, I can't find a satisfactory answer to the question.

I think we all have refrigerators because everyone on TV has one. I think we have TVs because everyone has one of those. I don't know why we don't have more time, better family relationships, more fun, and more love, but I am pretty sure it's all connected.

Why did we invade Iraq?

(After a year without the refrigerator, my wife found one that fit where the old refrigerator was, and we bought it, over my strenuous objection. I think refrigerators are silly and wasteful, and left to myself, I'd give ours up in an instant. The choice was between marriage and the refrigerator. The marriage won out, but only ever so barely.)

Not Eating Starts In The Grocery Store

America why are your libraries full of tears?
America when will you send your eggs to India?
I'm sick of your insane demands.
When can I go into the supermarket and buy what I
need with my good looks?
– Allen Ginsberg, *America*, 1956

If you don't have a refrigerator or any shelves, shopping for food so that you can eat intelligently is easy. You just don't buy anything that can spoil, which means you shop one day at a time. Otherwise, everything else you know about food shopping needs to be unlearned.

I can't tell you how many kids who are obviously overweight I take care of, but it is a lot. Each one has a mother. Part of my normal set of questions includes this one: "stay away from junk food?" Every kid answers the same way, with the same guilty shrug. Then I turn to the mother. "Who does the shopping?" I ask. The mother then almost always exhibits the same guilty shrug. "I can't help it," moms always say. "It's all my kids will eat."

"Will" is a funny word. No child has ever starved for lack of junk food. "I can't help it" is also a funny expression. When was the last time you saw a mother with a gun pointed to her head, being forced to buy junk food? Self, boundaries, psychology, marketing, anxiety, guilt, profit, and money all come into play when you walk into the supermarket, but not much thinking about why you are there survives the first aisle. When was the last time you walked into the supermarket, and walked out again with only one thing? When was the last time you walked into a supermarket, and walked out with only what you actually needed to eat to survive?

Even if you have a refrigerator, you can pretend you don't, and buy only a few items at a time. Cook only what you intend to eat that day. That way all the food you have will be fresh, you won't have to be throwing away spoiled food, and you won't have to look for packages that are buried beneath other packages which are buried beneath other packages, because there won't be any packages.

If you don't have extra calories in the house, you are much less likely to eat what you don't need.

If you don't have junk food in the house, then you can't eat it when you are home.

If you don't buy soda, you can't drink it. If you don't buy pasta, or potatoes, or rice, then you can't make pasta, potatoes or rice. If you buy only fresh vegetables, and lean meats, and fish, and fruit, then that's all you will cook and eat.

If you buy watermelon in the winter, people will look at you strangely, but it will be hard for you to carry much else, and when you think you are hungry, you'll eat watermelon, and not ice cream.

Practice walking in and out of the supermarket without buying anything. Do it four or five times. You won't destroy the gross domestic product by not buying what you don't need. It doesn't hurt.

Then practice not walking into the supermarket at all. For weeks at a time. Even for years.

There is nothing to fear but fear itself. And little to lose that we haven't lost already. And much to gain – like time, imagination, and hope - that we really need.

The Heck With 4 Food Groups. Kill The Starch. Stamp Out Greed.

Between 1985 and 2000, American food producers increased their output by 700 calories per person, to 3900 calories per person. During those years, the average caloric intake in the US went up by 300 to 400 calories. The bulk of that increase was from the consumption of foods made from corn, which increased 300 percent, and from wheat, which increased 150 percent. In 15 years!!![31]

Every plate, at every meal, at every table in every home and restaurant in America has the same appearance. Three items. Protein – meat or fish – vegetables, for complex carbohydrates, fiber and other nutrients, and starch, for energy, the holy trinity of eating in America. Where did this come from? Most of us remember hearing about the need for a balanced diet. I remember hearing about four food groups, and the need for a balanced diet, as I was growing up in the nineteen fifties and sixties, and always assumed that the whole concept was a government recommendation designed to insure good nutrition, so people would grow strong and resilient. The four food groups – milk, meats, vegetables and fruits, and breads and cereal - showed up on lots of posters and pictures that would be displayed in cafeterias and health classes across the country, and those food groups put a government approved, quasi-scientific stamp, on American eating. By indicating the number of servings a day of each food groups that Americans were supposed to eat, USDA made it clear that starch was king – four servings a day meant one serving at each meal, and one starch snack. The pictures of the plates on those posters and charts – one zone for meat, one for vegetables, and one for starch - imprinted the construction of meals on the brains of all Americans, so most of us can't conceptualize a meal that doesn't include potatoes, fries, or pasta, or rice. Purveyors of fast food capitalize on the ambiguity of potatoes – a vegetable that is also a starch, and purports to give you two groups in one item at each meal - the rise of French Fries.

(Some of us remember how Wonder Bread was supposed to "help build strong bodies 12 ways" – a slogan that always sounded scientific and focused on good nutrition, and still sounds so today, until you realized it was an attempt to sell sliced white bread, which is just a pre-sliced, homogenized, industrialized bread like product with added vitamins and minerals that come stuffed with preserva-

tives and wrapped in plastic. The sales pitch, about a product that is a major
source of unneeded calories delivered in a form that helps eliminate physical
work (the slicing!), makes you think that the calories in starch are needed to
build bodies, even though the only real nutritional value, in a country awash
in calories, was in the added vitamins and minerals. Those vitamins that could
come just as well from a "well balanced" diet built around vegetables and fruits
– or even from a simple daily vitamin.)

The notion of four food groups sounded like government propaganda to a country coming off two major wars, and to people accustomed, in the late forties and
early fifties, to regulations and recommendations from a government focused
on war economies, in a country trying to get the most effective use of limited
resources. So few people suspected that the four food groups, like most government recommendations about eating and nutrition, had significant food industry
input.

The notion of food groups to guide good eating dates to 1917, and, not surpris-
ingly, came from the US Department of Agriculture, and not the Department
of Health and Human Services, or even the National Institutes of Health. Over
the next 90 years, USDA grouping, and recommendations for amounts of each
group to eat in a day, ranged all over the map. We started with five food groups
in 1917, went to 12 food groups, dropped to 8 food groups, then to seven food
groups. Then, in the 1950s, we settled on the four food groups I remember,
stayed at 4 groups for 22 years – although one arm of USDA used 11 groups
to help people plan meals and food budgets while another arm of USDA was
using 4 groups; and went to 6 food groups in the dietary pyramid (which was
initially yanked from distribution as soon as it was released.[32]) During this period, "food already was overabundant in the United States, and already supplied
more than enough calories for the population." [33]

Why so many changing regulations? USDA groups, and occasional recommendations, were the regulatory and political equivalent of a food fight, with
each sector of the agricultural economy throwing their financial clout and political connections at one another, in the pursuit of a set of recommendations
that might increase their market share. They focused on the number and size of
servings suggested by the food groups, and fought viciously with one another,
and for the language "eat more of" their product at every opportunity. Sena-
tor George McGovern, presidential candidate in 1972 and chair of the Senate
Select Committee on Nutrition and Human Health, was defeated for re-election
in 1980, partly because he had offended the beef farming interests in South

32 Nestle, Marion. Food politics. Berkeley, The University of California Press, 2002. Pages 34- 66.
33 Nestle, Marion. Food politics. Berkeley, The University of California Press, 2002. p 34

Dakota when his hapless committee issued a report called Dietary Goals for the United States, a report that included the suggestion that Americans reduce fat to less than 30 percent of calories, which, though it was based on the best science available at the time, meant Americans would need to eat less beef. Good science is not always good business. "Eat less" of anything began a third rail of politics, a recommendation that no one in government could comfortably afford to make. With Conagra, General Foods, General Mills, Quaker Oats, and lots of congress people from farming states in the mix, no one in government would even look at eating less of a whole food group, which was also an icon of American culture. Remember "corn is as high as an elephants's eye?" and "amber waves of grain?"

Instead of just promoting "balanced" eating after food became plentiful in the US, the four food groups also provided a way to assure different kinds of food industrialists a seat at the table, or, they hoped, a seat at every table. In the case of starch – food products including or made from flour, potatoes, and rice - the food industrialists took a seat at a table which already had enough sitters, thank you very much.

It's a good bet that the inclusion of starch as the fourth food group is rooted in our history, not in our science. Before refrigeration, that is, prior to the nineteen twenties - less than 100 years ago - people depended on locally produced, and locally available foods. Fruits and vegetables in season. Meat, bought and consumed on the same day, just a few days after slaughter. Root crops from the root cellar. Preserved vegetables, to get you through the winter. And starches – wheat and wheat products, pasta, rice, and potatoes. Starches were magic energy sources because they could be easily stored without refrigeration. Starches were relatively easy to transport. And, with improvements in farming technologies and government subsidies, starches were efficient to produce and so could be sold cheaply. Of all the foods available to Americans at the turn of the 20th century, only starch was available reliably and inexpensively, which is what must have helped starch earn its place on the plate.

What's different of course, in the last 100 years, is the availability and cost of other foods, which happened together with the disappearance of manual work, and a likely drop in required daily calories. We just don't need the calories that starches contain. Protein is a good energy source, and also contains the amino acids that are necessary for muscle building and tissue repair. The complex carbohydrates found in vegetables are also a good energy source, and, because they break down slowly in the digestive system, cause fewer swings in blood sugar and insulin levels, and less metabolic chaos. Vegetables also have many other needed nutrients, and no preservatives or extra ingredients. In 2009, fresh vegetables, meats, and fish are available year round, even to those of us who don't have a refrigerator and shop daily. With many of us having plenty of energy stores, the four food group meal is no longer necessary. Simply put, there is no need to include a starch in every meal, since all starch adds is calories. There may be no need for starch at all.

That won't please the sugar lobby, the corn lobby, the wheat lobby, and the agribusiness oligarchs. But guess why corn syrup and corn starch and sugar are inexpensive, and find their way into almost all processed foods? Because starches, are, by and large, heavily subsidized.

We will spend $190 billion on farm subsidies by 2012, much of which goes to encouraging farmers of corn and wheat to grow more corn and wheat, and the prices of both commodities are so low that we've created whole industries that convert them to other usable products, like ethanol and high fructose corn syrup, each with their own controversial environmental and health impacts.[34] The presence of so much excess starch in the American economy means constant advocacy, by their producers, processors, and marketers, for Americans to consume more starch.

What a wonderful world we have created! We subsidize many starches, because of the profit motive. Subsidized corn starch and fructose gets into lots of foods, making it inexpensive. We promote those foods in the marketplace and even in the government's nutritional messaging, and we are shocked, shocked, when we discover we have an obese population with too much diabetes, heart disease, stroke, and cancer. Then we start doing surgery on the people who weigh too much, doling out expensive drugs to the millions of diabetics, placing stents in a zillion hearts, and use more medicine to bring down the cholesterol of our overweight people, and we are shocked, shocked, when our medical spending goes out of control, and cripples our economy, so we have nothing left to spend on education, housing and the environment, the programs most likely to make the population healthy and happy.

It turns out to be easy to eliminate starch from your diet, once you understand there is no need for it to be there. You can make dinner with just chicken, meat or fish, a fresh or cooked vegetable, and a salad. You don't really need the pasta or rice – it's just a habit. You won't feel hungry if you don't have home fries for breakfast. You don't need breakfast cereal or even breakfast bars in the morning. Fruit, or salad will do just fine. You don't need toast or bagels or

34 Fields S. The Fat of the Land: Do Agricultural Subsidies Foster Poor Health? Environmental Health Perspectives Volume 112, Number 14, October 2004

English muffins in the morning either. You don't have to stop for donuts – fruit or a cup of coffee works beautifully. There is no nutritional value in cookies, coffee cake or candy bars. And potato or corn chips? Think of how many cravings, and how much eating has been produced by people who have something to sell.

I'll say it again. It is humanly possible to have a plate without a starch on it. Just like no kid ever died from lack of junk food, no otherwise healthy American of any age, who has a BMI of 20 or greater, ever died from not eating starch. The opposite is probably true – it is starch that is killing us. You can get all the energy you need from protein and complex carbohydrate, which is plentiful in the American diet. There is no imaginable adverse health effect from eliminating starch in your diet. There is no need for starch to be a food group any more. Like smoking cigarettes, starch is an American habit that turned out to be bad for us, one we should just give up, now that we know it is harmful, and despite the adverse economic effect giving up starch will have on the people who make money producing and marketing it.

Sure, you won't get the warm, relaxed buzz many people get after eating too much potatoes or rice at the end of the day, but is over-consumption really the best way to combat stress? Maybe the best way to combat stress is to prevent it – to understand the vicious cycle we have created for ourselves – eat more, buy more, pay more, need to exercise more, need to doctor more, need to work more, sleep less, worry more – and unwind that cycle, by understanding that we are all eating and doing too much, that can does not mean should, that want does not mean have, that someone else's profit does not have to be your loss.

We have met the enemy and he is us.

Give up starch, and stamp out greed.

Save Time And Money. Eat Less.

One of the hidden advantages to eating less is that you'll save money. Maybe.
Depends on how much you drop back, and what you choose to eat.

Say you are eating 2000 calories a day, when you really need 1200, and you are
exercising an hour a day to try to keep up with your eating, which means you
are probably still gaining weight, and you drop back to 1200 calories. You've
shed 800 calories a day, or 40 percent of your caloric intake, and you can get
your whole family to do the same.

According to the Economic Research Service of the USDA, the average annual
food cost per person in 2007 was $1935 at home plus $1842 away from home
for total of $3777 per person per year.[35] Thus a family of 4 spends $15,108 for
food. If you can reduce your calories by just 20 percent, you'll save $3000 per
year. If you can reduce your calories by 40 percent, you'll save $6000 per year.
Or more. Because over time you'll save much more on what you had to spend
on treatment for health problems caused by obesity. And you'll have more time
for work or relaxation. If you have to exercise an extra hour a day to burn the
calories that you are eating that you don't need, then you have an extra hour a
day to spend as you want, a significant savings.

(Talk about excess. There's lots of good evidence that between 1985 and 2000,
Americans started eating an extra 300 calories a day, almost all from corn and
wheat products, and the nation's food industry started producing an extra 700
calories a day.[36] Did it occur to anyone to eat less? No. Instead, we, the nation,
and the nation's doctors, started recommending more exercise, so people from
all walks of life started getting up at 5 am to go work out, and started spending lots of money on exercise machines and gym memberships. Which meant
everyone had to work harder and spend more time away from home to do the
exercise and pay for the cost of doing it. Get the cycle? Agribusiness emerges,
and convinces Congress to give more subsidies to corn and wheat growers, who
grow more corn and wheat, making it inexpensive. Everyone eats more, and
gains weight. People start getting sick, because they eat more, and gain weight.
The cost of health insurance goes up, because people get sick from eating too
much, and everyone has to work harder to pay for their health care. Everyone

35 http://www.ers.usda.gov/Briefing/CPIFoodAndExpenditures/Data/table15.htm. 12/11/2008 9:15 AM
36 http://www.ers.usda.gov/publications/FoodReview/DEC2002/frvol25i3a.pdf. 12/11/2008 9:30 AM

starts exercising more, and spending more time away from home to exercise. We all get ornery, and then we invade Iraq. Who is the enemy? Al-Qaida, or us, or both?)

Truth be told, there's no guarantee you'll save money if you eat less, because people smart enough to eat less are also smart enough to choose better foods, and over the last few years, it's the better foods, particularly fresh fruits and vegetables, that have become more expensive, while subsidized starch prices have stayed stable or declined. You'll probably spend more time shopping, if you buy what you eat daily. So if you eat less but you improve the quality of the food you eat, you might not save as much. But you might, by stopping at farm stands and farmer's markets, start supporting local agriculture and the local economy, in a way you might not be doing now. And you might start growing some of your own food. And you might see and talk to people you hadn't talked to before, or don't see much. So you might not save that much cash money right away, but you just might be helping to make a better life for everyone, which is worth all the money in the world.

One quick disclaimer: at 1200 calories, you might not get the recommended amounts of vitamins and minerals you get from a 2500 calorie or 2000 calorie diet, which are used as the basis to compute those recommended amounts. On the other hand, if you improve the quality and diversity of your food, you just might get more of those vitamins and minerals than you are getting now. The recommended daily allowances were also not based on a varied diet with lots of fruits and vegetables. I wouldn't worry about it. One of the things I learned from taking care of children is not to worry about what a child eats – there is plenty of evidence that suggests, left to themselves over time, children seek out the foods that contain the nutrients they need, and in the correct amounts. My guess is that if you eat a good varied diet, focused on fruits and vegetables, you'll get what you need, and your own preferences will steer you to address any short term deficiencies. In 25 years of practice, I can count on the fingers of one hand the number of people I saw who suffered from the consequences of nutritional deficiencies, and those were almost all menstruating women who developed iron deficiency, something you can usually prevent by eating lots of green leafy vegetables. The risks of eating 2500 calories a day, and dealing with the health, psychological, and social consequences of eating that way and living in that culture over time, far outweigh any potential nutritional deficiencies that might come from eating a thoughtful diet.

If It's Not There, You Won't Eat It. If It's There, You Will.

In a wonderful, human, funny, and insightful book called Mindless Eating, Brian Wansink Ph.D., whose training is in marketing but who is expert at what might be called eating psychology, explores the science about what makes people eat, and what makes people not eat, and what makes people stop eating once they start.[37]

What makes people eat? Essentially everything. There are zillions of cues to eat - anxiety, proximity, portion size, setting, situation, color, texture, status - all unrelated to caloric need, that stimulate both eating and the perception of pleasure from eating, which also appears to have little to do with what and how much food people actually eat.

What makes people not eat? Essentially nothing. Like the 2000 Year Old Man's discovery of women, if there is food present, people will eat it.

What makes people stop eating? Also essentially nothing. We eat until the food is gone. Your stomach, says Wansink, can't count, and apparently your brain can't count either. This was a great nutritional strategy from our past, when food was scarce and we needed to capture every available calorie to prevent starvation, but in a world where food is plentiful, it is causing us to eat ourselves to death. There are lots of cues to tell us to eat. But there are almost no cues to tell us to stop eating. We are terrible at estimating portion size, particularly when portions are larger; we are terrible at remembering how much we just ate, so we keep eating, and we are worse at estimating how many calories there are in what we are eating.

Wansink describes a wonderful study he conducted, meant to test the relative contribution of taste and of setting and portion size in determining what, and how much people will eat. They provided free popcorn (and a free soft drink!) to a theatre full of moviegoers at a 1:05 pm Saturday matinee, right after most people would have had lunch. The popcorn came in two sizes – medium, and large - but both sized containers were actually so large that it was unlikely any one person would finish all the popcorn in the container.

---

37 Wansink, Brian. Mindless Eating. New York: Bantam Books, 2006.

But there was one catch. The popcorn was 5 days old, and was as stale as styrofoam.

A few people noticed, and went to the refreshment stand and asked for their money back (pretty amazing, since the popcorn was free). But most people ate most of what was in the container they had been given, a little at a time. And even more amazing, the people who had been given the larger size container ate more of the stale popcorn – an average of 173 more calories of stale popcorn.

There was nothing telling people not to eat. The bigger the package, the more they ate.

We can't not eat. We are programmed to eat, and into that programming, American Agribusiness has poured 3900 calories of food per person per day into a population that needs, my guess is, 1000 to 1200 - but no more than 1500 calories a day. Remember the seven fat cows and the seven lean cows? We are living in the time of seven fat cows, and our problem is how to make them lean again, so they don't explode, or get eaten themselves.

So here are suggestions about not eating, some from Wansink, and some from others, that come from the realization that the only way normal humans won't eat is if they can't get, or have a hard time getting at, food.

1. Don't leave food out. If you walk by it, you will eat it.
2. Don't save leftovers. (A corollary to kill you refrigerator. Killing your refrigerator is cheaper, but not having or saving leftovers works almost as well.)
3. Put everything you eat on a plate.
4. Don't eat alone. You didn't need the calories anyway.
5. Don't eat standing up.
6. Trash your dinner plates. Use only salad plates, which are smaller.
7. Don't bring leftovers home from restaurants.
8. Don't eat until you've exercised.
9. Taste, but don't inhale.

Part V - Ok, But What *Can* I Eat?

The Joy Of Eating

But food tastes good, and it is comfort and joy. There's nothing better than a good meal, and a glass of good wine, with old friends.

How true.

The eater's dilemma. Food tastes good. Great eating is its own reward. It's a great reason to be with people you love. But you don't need the calories.

Truth: great food, like true love, is one of life's transcendent pleasures, something you should never deny yourself in your time on this earth. But how often does true love last?

But. (Sorry, reality intervening.) How often is what you eat great food – really, truly, transcendent overwhelming saturation of the senses? And how often do you go someplace hoping for that transcendent experience, and find thoughtful, competent cooking – or worse – and eat too damn much anyway, because it is there?

So, a way to eat, mindful that you don't need many calories, and mindful that you carry a few months of energy stores with you all the time, and that your brain is programmed to eat what's put in front of you and to go back for seconds.

Taste everything, eat little. With each mouthful, ask yourself the question: is this a transcendent sensory moment? If it's not, stop - you tasted and that was all you need – don't finish what's on your plate, and don't ask for more. If it is, eat it all, and savor each bite and each moment. Drink deep. Life is short – too short to waste on bad food and mediocre experiences.

The good news is, there aren't that many transcendent sensory moments in eating, so your risk of eating too much, if you can stick to this principle, is minimal – and why be afraid to live just because American Agribusiness overproduces the wrong things? Their profit doesn't have to be your loss.

Share. If you share meals with people you love, you get to find out if something is that transcendent sensory moment, you get to be with people you love, and you aren't taking in calories you didn't need. Everyone wins. (Except perhaps the restaurant industry, because you ordered and spent less.)

Try new things. Life is short.

Drink things you love when you are thirsty. Eat low calorie things you love when you have to eat something. Remember, you need enough sodium to replace what you lose every day.

Taste everything. Share. The Zero Calorie Diet tells us what to eat, and what not to eat, and how much we each really need. Knowing what to eat, and what not to eat, and how much we each really need, is something like knowing how to live.

We didn't have to invade Iraq. There are better ways to build democracy around the world than bombs and missiles. We can feed the world, and bring schools and health centers, as a place to start. Just because we are programmed to eat, we can learn to eat intelligently before eating kills us, and everyone else – before we all explode.

The Greater Than Zero Calorie Diet

What to eat? Not much. First drink if you want to, then eat if you have to.

The advice I'm going to give is unconventional, particularly in a world that has worked to create low cost, high calorie, low fat and salt snacks, all in fancy wrappers.

I'd eat foods that are low in calories, high in salt and not wrapped in plastic. I'd forget about fat. I just wouldn't eat much.

Let's think about the fat part first. Worries about the fat in diet were based on a 2500 calorie diet. On 1200 calories, you don't get enough fat to do you any harm, unless that's all you eat. It's still worth while avoiding fried foods, whole milk products, and lots of eggs – but if I had chickens, which I do, and they laid eggs, which they do, I'd eat the eggs, which I do. You'll burn the fat taking care of the chickens, and if you are eating 1200 calories a day and doing lots of real physical work, the fat in eggs isn't likely to hurt you. (I wouldn't eat eggs if I were totally sedentary, 1200 calorie diet or not.)

The salt part. I'd eat foods that have a lot of salt, just not much of them, so I'd get 1.5 grams of sodium a day, for two weeks after dropping my caloric intake, and then I'd stop. Pickles, deli meats and beef jerky fit the bill, as do most soups. The other option is to salt lower salt foods, like vegetables. No need to go nuts about this, but it will help you tolerate the change in diet, as long as you drink enough. I might not do this if I had high blood pressure, or, since only about 1/3 of people have high blood pressure that gets worse with a little salt, I might do it anyway, and use a home blood pressure machine to take my blood pressure once a day, to make sure it stays in control.

But mostly, I'd concentrate on low calorie foods, like fruits and vegetables. Once you are drinking and taking enough salt, the need to feel full seems to go away, so vegetables work well at mealtimes. Sweet potatoes, broccoli, corn, carrots, beans, squash, cucumbers, tomatoes, lettuce – as my son says, it's all good. You get different amounts of protein, complex carbohydrate, and many other nutrients, and in general they are not contaminated with preservatives and dyes.

Meats? Fine in small amounts. When I started making lots of vegetables and salads, I dropped our meat consumption to 4 ounces in a portion, and it works fine. We eat meat twice a week. Just not very much.

Fish? Same as meat. We try to eat it once a week. Small portions – 4-6 ounces per person.

Fruit? Like vegetables. Okay to eat after drinking something.

Starch? Completely unnecessary. There is adequate carbohydrate in vegetables and fruits.

What does a meal look like?

Breakfast is fruit and 2 cups of tea of coffee, with midmorning tea or a cup or watermelon when I get bored.

Lunch is deli meat or beef, venison, salmon, elk, buffalo, reindeer or even tofu jerky, often with a cup of bouillon, and 2 glasses of water. No bread, which means eating the meat with one's fingers. The combination of the protein from the meat and the salt from the meat or the bouillon, and the water, is filling and brings me back to life after a morning of working hard, inside or out.

Dinner is a salad, a pickle, a slice of watermelon, and 4 to 6 ounces of meat or fish, and vegetables – often lightly cooked, often cooked in wine. Sometimes beans or rice and beans. Lots to drink. We get variation in what we eat by eating different vegetables, and preparing the different vegetables differently.

When should you eat?

First, I'm unconvinced by the three-meals-a-day argument. There is evidence in favor of breakfast. You get a minor release of growth hormone if you eat breakfast, and in general, growth hormone is a good thing, but I'm not sure eating in the morning really matters. Remember, the three meals a day concept comes from the early sixties, when the US caloric intake had just become secure. It was the early days of agribusiness, when food producers had everything to gain if you ate more calories, and there were cereal makers whose bottom lines depended on your whole family sitting down to breakfast every day, a concept I remember myself, and I've seen on TV, but haven't encountered in real life since 1965 or so, perhaps because everyone is out exercising to burn off the extra calories they are eating.

The three-meal-a-day concept dated from a time when energy sources were thought important, and energy was an issue, because most people were still lean. But we haven't had an issue with energy availability in 25 years. Most of us have adequate energy stores to get through the day, even the week and the month, so packing in more energy, which will end up stored as fat, doesn't really seem necessary. As a social experience, breakfast is a fine idea. As a nutritional experience, I'm not sure it matters.

Likewise lunch. The real value of lunch is that it lets people take some time from working to connect with each other, and for thinking and dreaming. A little fluid, and a little protein, go a long way.

Dinner is a time for people to get together, and also eat. Its major focus should be the time spent together, and the taste – but not the amount - of the food that gets eaten.

Of note, Americans now consume about half of our calories outside the home. That fact presents challenges and opportunities. The major challenge is the ability to control portion size and food quality when you eat out. The major opportunity is the opportunity of using food to change your relationships with friends. Share meals. Eat salads or soups. Don't get suckered by large portions – you don't need them anyway. (One wonders how much eating away from home occurs because Americans are out working longer to pay for our extra calories, to pay for the exercising we have to do to deal with the weight we put on from eating the extra calories, and the medical expenses we run up because of the weight.)

Food That Can Help You Not Eat

An Ode to Watermelon

I think watermelon is nature's perfect food for life in 2010. I'm sure some-one will someday do a controlled standardized double-blind crossover trial and prove that watermelon is worse than eating only beef fat, but until they do, and feed a watermelon a week to a thousand people for 2 years, I'm going to think watermelon is what we should eat.

Here's why: 48 calories a cup. Lots of fluid. Lots of potassium. Lots of lycopenes – probably more than any other food. (Lycopenes are supposed to prevent cancer, though I always wonder how much meaning theories about things like lycopenes actually have, because cancer is a disease with many dif-ferent causes, the most significant of which is aging. Remember, everyone dies of something, and if heart disease and lung disease don't get your, cancer will.) Eighteen percent of the Daily Value for Vitamin A. Twenty-one percent of the Daily Value for Vitamin C. Lesser amounts of the B vitamins, decent calcium. No fat to speak of. Sugar, but as complex, not simple carbohydrate. Not much sodium, but a little.

You can get watermelon year round. It doubles in price during the fall and win-ter months, but it still costs less, per pound, than any other fruit.

But here's its real value. Relative rates. If you are eating watermelon, which has relatively few calories per cup, it's like drinking because of its fluid content (each cup has about 150 milliliters of water, or more than half a cup of fluid, so it removes one of the stimuli to drink and eat) and it means you are not eat-ing something else, which is likely to have more calories for the same volume. If you eat one cup of watermelon, and take in 48 calories, that's much better for you then eating 1 cup of ice cream, which gives you 400 calories, or one 8 ounce bag of potato chips, which has 1272 calories, and in fact, probably more (since no one seems to be able to eat just one). One cup of watermelon has less calories than about any food I can think of, except celery, which has less than 15 calories per cup but doesn't taste anywhere near as good, and pickles, which have only 5 calories each, but have way too much salt to eat more than five a day.

You can eat a cup of watermelon an hour for a whole ten hour work day and still have enough calories left over to eat a decent dinner – and that's like drinking 6 cups of your 12 to 15 cups of water a day.

Who needs junk food?

Surimi Sutra

Surimi is the one excuse for the industrialization of food that I can think of. It is processed fish, mostly pollack or whiting, with flavorings and coloring to make it taste like crab or lobster. It doesn't quite taste like either, but because they use sweeteners, it is quite good, with the best surimi tasting fine on its own (though not quite as good as lobster or crab – but then, surimi is much easier to eat).

80 calories per 4 ounce serving. 320 milligrams of sodium. No fat. Decent protein. Like any other fish, but a little less expensive, and easily available. Surimi is a great protein source, easily made part of a salad or served with rice and beans, or eaten on its own.

There just isn't a better protein source. Chicken has twice as many calories for the same volume, and more fat.

All praise Beef Jerky

Beef, turkey, elk, venison, buffalo and salmon jerky are great foods. Mostly protein and high in sodium, low in fat, they are perfect to use for a midday lunch or snack, as long as you limit the amount to an ounce or two. Native Americans carried jerky when they went hunting, because it was light weight, didn't spoil, and contained enough energy to power hard work.

Some jerky is preserved with sodium nitrate, which should be viewed with caution. Sodium nitrate has an association with cancers of the GI tract, and recently was found to have an association with pancreatic cancer in one study, though the risk of pancreatic cancer is low from a population perspective, which makes it easy to claim an increase in a population that might only be due to chance or some other variable. I'm generally suspicious of studies which link a nutrient or chemical to cancer, unless there is overwhelming impressive evidence from many studies, and sodium nitrate as a carcinogen doesn't pass that test, in part because sodium nitrate is also found in vegetables, which makes it hard to figure out what is actually causing the cancers when they occur. But since there is lots of jerky made without nitrates available, using nitrate free jerky is a perfectly reasonable thing to do.

If jerky could sustain our ancestors on a three day hunt, it can probably sustain us, with lots of fluid, during a 10 hour work day, as we try to eat less.

Hallelujah Pickles

Pickles are a source of sodium which put a little spice in daily eating. Five calories each, 250 to 350 milligrams of sodium, pickles will help you maintain your blood volume if you drink fluid the same day you eat them. One with dinner makes a salad more zesty. There are lots of kinds, so you can vary things. They work.

The Ballad of Bouillon

Bouillon is there for the salt. Short term as you switch to eating less calories, but a great warm food in the middle of the day when you are trying to control your day time calories and want your brain to work. 500 to 1300 milligrams of sodium per cup. Ten calories. Nothing else like it.

The Zero Calorie Diet Lite

There's another way to eat less, think about what you do, and still live in the modern world.

Regular intermittent one day fasting.

That is, you fast every other day, or every third day, or once a week.

You do The Zero Calorie Diet, but only one day at a time.

Same basic construction – no calories, supplement fluid, replace sodium.

The good news is that The Zero Calorie Diet Lite is relatively easy to do. It's not hard to go a day without eating, particularly if you replace fluid and sodium. You get the same kind of control over your eating, and feel a new sense of balance in your life, as you realize that no one and nothing, no advertisement, no anxiety, no government recommendation, can make you do what you don't need to do. The Zero Calorie Diet Lite helps you balance the demands of a busy world, to compensate for the days you are traveling, or the days when there is just too much food around – the family celebration, the holiday season, or the meeting or conference, when you find you ate too much at the breaks, trying to stay awake.

The better news is that there is very early experimental evidence supporting the use of The Zero Calorie Diet Lite. Though most of the work reported is from animal studies, it appears that alternate day fasts help lower cholesterol, raise HDL (or good cholesterol), lower heart rate, and may lower blood pressure. In animals, alternate day fasting may slow the rate of growth of certain cell lines, which, conceivably, might help slow or prevent cancer.[38]

The major advantage of The Zero Calorie Diet Lite is how it helps you think about eating and not eating. It's another way to help you remember that what counts is not what you eat, or do, in a day. It's what you eat, or do, in your life, one day at a time.

---

38 Varady KA, Hellerstein MK. Alternate-day fasting and chronic disease prevention: a review of human and animal trials. Am J Clin Nutr. 2007 Jul;86(1):7-13

But, like The Zero Calorie Diet, the reason for doing The Zero Calorie Diet Lite is not to help you live forever. It's there to help you think, and to give you a platform from which to see how things are connected to what you choose to do, or not do, every day of your life.

Part VI - Work

> # Physical Work Is Like Not Eating, Only Different. Police The Area. Pack Out Your Trash. Burn What You Eat.

First, some random facts about burning calories.

The first critical idea is that your body will burn calories by breaking down body tissues once your energy needs are greater than your energy intake, and that you don't get to control which body tissues the body breaks down.

When your energy needs are greater than your energy intake, the first thing your body does is burn a stored form of glucose, called glycogen, that is stored in the liver and in muscle. Once it goes through the glycogen (which usually takes 8 to 12 hours), the body starts to break down tissues, which it needs to make glucose, a fuel the brain depends upon, and, at the same time, the body starts to burn fat. Initially, the body breaks down tissues faster than it burns fat, but by the end of 2 weeks, the body is getting 90 percent of its energy requirements from fat, and it tends to leave the muscles alone, though it always needs to break down some muscle, because it just can't make enough energy to supply the brain from fat alone.

What tissues does the body break down, and in what order? We know that we stop making digestive enzymes early, which makes sense, because there is nothing to digest. The muscle proteins start to break down at a high rate, but that rate slows, but doesn't vanish, once the body starts using fat for energy.

Are all muscles broken down at the same rate? No one knows. In the early protein sparing fasts of the late 1970s, it was believed that heart muscle was broken down at the same rate as other muscles, and that breakdown caused the high rate of sudden death. But now there is evidence suggesting that heart muscle is preserved during fasting. A recent study (interestingly enough, from Cleveland, where the initial work on protein sparing fasts was done) suggests that heart muscle building is preserved during periods of calorie restriction.[39]

---

39 Yuan CL, Sharma N, Gilge DA, Stanley WC, Li Y, Hatzoglou M, Previs SF. Preserved protein synthesis in the heart in response to acute fasting and chronic food restriction despite reductions in liver and skeletal muscle. Am J Physiol Endocrinol Metab. 2008 Jul;295(1):E216-22. Epub 2008 Apr 29

What is unknown is the role of exercise. We know that exercise, that the use of a muscle, is the major signal that stimulates the muscle's getting larger and stronger. What we don't know is what happens to a muscle when exercise occurs during fasting or other times of calorie restriction. On the one hand, the body is trying to break muscles down, to use the protein scavenged from the muscle as an energy source for the brain. On the other hand, exercising muscle stimulates that same muscle to grow larger and stronger, perhaps using the breakdown products of fat as an energy source for muscle as well as brain.

There are two interesting lessons from this. The first, not proven, may be that exercising during a fast may prevent sudden cardiac deaths from fasting, because it preserves cardiac muscle. The second lesson, perhaps more interesting for people who are trying to improve their body's condition, is that the impact of weight loss on parts of the body is unpredictable, but exercise, during periods of calorie restriction, will improve the tone of the body overall. That is, if you have reduced your intake of calories, you just can't predict how it is going to make you look, particularly if you don't exercise. Say you want to lose a flabby gut and you just reduce your intake of calories. The gut may stay where it is for a very long time – but you may see your neck size shrink and your legs thin and even find lost cheekbones again, long before you see your waist shrink, and no particular exercise will change that. What exercise can do, however, is help you build the size and power of the muscles you use during exercise. If you are running (an exercise I don't usually recommend, because it causes people to wear out their knees), your legs will get powerful and strong. If you are splitting wood, your back and arms will get powerful and strong, but your gut may shrink more slowly then you expect. The overall lesson: neither fasting nor calorie restriction alone will create a Madison Avenue body. Even exercise, which will help you feel better and get stronger, is unlikely to change either your body or your life in a predictable way. So getting a Madison Avenue body is probably not reason enough to change your life, if getting a Madison Avenue body is what you want to achieve.

Is it smart to eat an extra 300 calories a day, and then exercise an hour to burn them off? That's what many Americans – the one third of us who aren't gaining weight - are doing. (Many others are trying and failing. We are much better at eating the extra three hundred calories than we are at doing an hour of exercise to burn off those extra calories.) When you eat extra and exercise extra, you stay in good cardiovascular shape, and keep your risk of diabetes and heart disease from growing with your extra calorie intake. Many people who exercise stay mentally alert.

But. But. But. Big Bill Haywood, of the IWW used to say, "When one man has a dollar he didn't work for, some other man worked for a dollar he didn't get."

Which is to say, when one of us takes in three hundred calories we didn't need, someone else, somewhere around the world, needed three hundred calories he or she didn't get. Or, when one of us takes in three hundred calories we didn't need, we used a little bit of the planet's energy reserves that we might have saved for future generations or hard times, and probably made global warming a little worse. On a personal level, is it worth it to eat an extra bowl of ice cream each night, and then have to add a hour of exercise to your life, to say nothing of getting to and from your preferred method of exercise? Is it worth working harder to pay for the extra 300 hundred calories, and then harder yet, to pay for the gym membership and to afford the time it takes to go to the gym?

You can build physical work into your life, and just skip the extra three hundred calories, and stay in shape just living your life. Garden, clean your own house, split wood, bicycle for joy or to work.

Listen.

Can does not mean should.

Want does not mean need.

Lean.

As a people, we have been overwhelmed by our appetites, and have overwhelmed the rest of the world with our bearing. Technology gave us the means to do things that were beyond our wildest dreams – to be in space, to communicate instantly around the globe, to travel, to control the environment – and to wreak unimaginable destruction on the planet and on each other.

Our bodies drive us to eat, and we have trouble not eating. Put an extra 300 or 400 calories in front of us, and we eat those 300 or 400 calories, whether we need them or not.

It's when we don't eat that we are listening.

The Zero Calorie Diet teaches you that you don't have to eat much, which means there is plenty of time to listen, to love, to labor and to bless our time on this earth.

Appendix

Formulae To Calculate Caloric Need

There are many formulae for estimating your daily caloric expenditure. Three are given here, but there are lots of others, and people have been arguing over which is more accurate for decades. It's a silly argument.

The problem with using these formulae is that they are estimates which are based on measurements of oxygen use, not direct measurements of how many calories you actually burned in a day, a measurement which is absurdly difficult to make. The problem with any estimate is that there are so many variables involved in actually determining how many calories you burn in a day – metabolic efficiency, activity, ambient temperature, emotional stress (which influences basic metabolic rate), how much you are eating, when you last ate, and what you have recently eaten, even how well you are sleeping.

So the only real measure of your caloric consumption is your weight. If your weight is going up over the course of a week, month, or year, you took in more calories than you burned. If your weight is going down over the course of a week, month or year, then you burned more calories than you took in. The longer period of time you use as a comparison, the more accurate your measurement is, because there are fairly significant day to day fluctuations in weight that result from when you last ate, when you last drank, and when you last used the toilet.

So obsessing over the numbers isn't really going to help you understand how much to eat or not eat. Only thinking matters, thinking about eating, nutrition, work, responsibility and relationships.

The Harris Benedict Equation

English BMR Formula
Women: BMR = 655 + (4.35 x weight in pounds) + (4.7 x height in inches) - (4.7 x age in years)
Men: BMR = 66 + (6.23 x weight in pounds) + (12.7 x height in inches) - (6.8 x age in year)
Metric BMR Formula Women: BMR = 655 + (9.6 x weight in kilos) + (1.8 x height in cm) - (4.7 x age in years)
Men: BMR = 66 + (13.7 x weight in kilos) + (5 x height in cm) - (6.8 x age in years)[1]

But Harris Benedict over predicts BMR by 15 percent in modern populations.[2]

The Mifflin-St Jeor Equation

Male: BMR = 10×weight + 6.25×height - 5×age + 5
Female: BMR = 10×weight + 6.25×height - 5×age - 161
These equations require the weight in kilograms, the height in centimeters, and the age in years.[3][4]

The Katch-McArdle Equation

The Katch-McArdle formula based on lean body mass:
BMR = 370 + (9.79759519 X Lean Mass in pounds)
The Katch –Mcardle formula may be more accurate for athletes, or people whose weight is close to their lean body mass.[5]

1 Harris J, Benedict F (1918). A Biometric Study of Human Basal Metabolism. Proc Sci U S a 4 (12): 370–3. doi:10.1073/pnas.4.12.370. PMID 16576330
2 http://www.adaevidencelibrary.com/worksheet.cfm?worksheet_id=250857 12/22/2008 10:36 AM
3 MD Mifflin, ST St Jeor, LA Hill, BJ Scott, SA Daugherty and YO Koh. A new predictive equation for resting energy expenditure in healthy individuals. American Journal of Clinical Nutrition, Vol 51, 241-247 (1990)
4 Frankenfield,D Roth-Yousey, L Compher C. Comparison of Predictive Equations for Resting Metabolic Rate in Healthy Nonobese and Obese Adults: A Systematic Review. J Am Diet Assoc Volume 105, Issue 5, Pages 775-789 (May 2005)
5 Katch, Frank, Katch, Victor, McArdle, William. Exercise Physiology: Energy, Nutrition, and Human Performance, 4th edition. Williams & Wilkins, 1996.

Improving The Accuracy of The Equations

To better estimate daily calorie needs, multiply the BMR by the appropriate activity factor, which gives you an estimate of total energy expenditure, as follows:

- 1.200 = sedentary (little or no exercise)
- 1.375 = lightly active (light exercise/sports 1-3 days/week)
- 1.550 = moderately active (moderate exercise/sports 3-5 days/week)
- 1.725 = very active (hard exercise/sports 6-7 days a week)
- 1.900 = extra active (very hard exercise/sports and physical job)

Body Mass Index Chart

To use the table, find the appropriate height in the left-hand column labeled Height. Move across to a given weight (in pounds). The number at the top of the column is the BMI at that height and weight. Pounds have been rounded off.

BMI	19	20	21	22	23	24	25	26	27
Height (inches)		Body Weight (pounds)							
58	91	96	100	105	110	115	119	124	129
59	94	99	104	109	114	119	124	128	133
60	97	102	107	112	118	123	128	133	138
61	100	106	111	116	122	127	132	137	143
62	104	109	115	120	126	131	136	142	147
63	107	113	118	124	130	135	141	146	152
64	110	116	122	128	134	140	145	151	157
65	114	120	126	132	138	144	150	156	162
66	118	124	130	136	142	148	155	161	167
67	121	127	134	140	146	153	159	166	172
68	125	131	138	144	151	158	164	171	177
69	128	135	142	149	155	162	169	176	182
70	132	139	146	153	160	167	174	181	188
71	136	143	150	157	165	172	179	186	193
72	140	147	154	162	169	177	184	191	199
73	144	151	159	166	174	182	189	197	204
74	148	155	163	171	179	186	194	202	210
75	152	160	168	176	184	192	200	208	216
76	156	164	172	180	189	197	205	213	221

http://www.nhlbi.nih.gov/guidelines/obesity/bmi_tbl.htm

28	29	30	31	32	33	34	35
134	138	143	148	153	158	162	167
138	143	148	153	158	163	168	173
143	148	153	158	163	168	174	179
148	153	158	164	169	174	180	185
153	158	164	169	175	180	186	191
158	163	169	175	180	186	191	197
163	169	174	180	186	192	197	204
168	174	180	186	192	198	204	210
173	179	186	192	198	204	210	216
178	185	191	198	204	211	217	223
184	190	197	203	210	216	223	230
189	196	203	209	216	223	230	236
195	202	209	216	222	229	236	243
200	208	215	222	229	236	243	250
206	213	221	228	235	242	250	258
212	219	227	235	242	250	257	265
218	225	233	241	249	256	264	272
224	232	240	248	256	264	272	279
230	238	246	254	263	271	279	287

Useful Links

For the Calculation of Basal Metabolic Rate (BMR)

http://www.calculatorslive.com/BMR-Calculator.aspx

http://www.nhlbi.nih.gov/guidelines/obesity/bmi_tbl.htm

The Sodium Content of Foods

http://www.ars.usda.gov/SP2UserFiles/Place/12354500/Data/SR22/nutrlist/sr22a307.pdf

The Caloric Content of Foods

http://www.ars.usda.gov/SP2UserFiles/Place/12354500/Data/SR22/nutrlist/sr22a208.pdf

Bibliography

Institute of Medicine. Daily Reference Guides: Water, Potassium, Sodium, Chloride an Sulfate. National Academies Press, 2004.

Nestle, Marion. Food Politics. Berkeley, The University of California Press, 2002.

Pollan, Michael. In Defense of Food - an eater's manifesto. New York: The Penguin Press, 2008

Wansink, Brian. Mindless Eating. New York: Bantam Books, 2006